THE TASTE OF THE CARIBBEAN CUISINE

By

Chef Liline

MY MODERN
CARIBBEAN KITCHEN

70+ Fresh Takes On Island Favorites

Darline Dorcely "The Chef"

TABLE OF CONTENTS

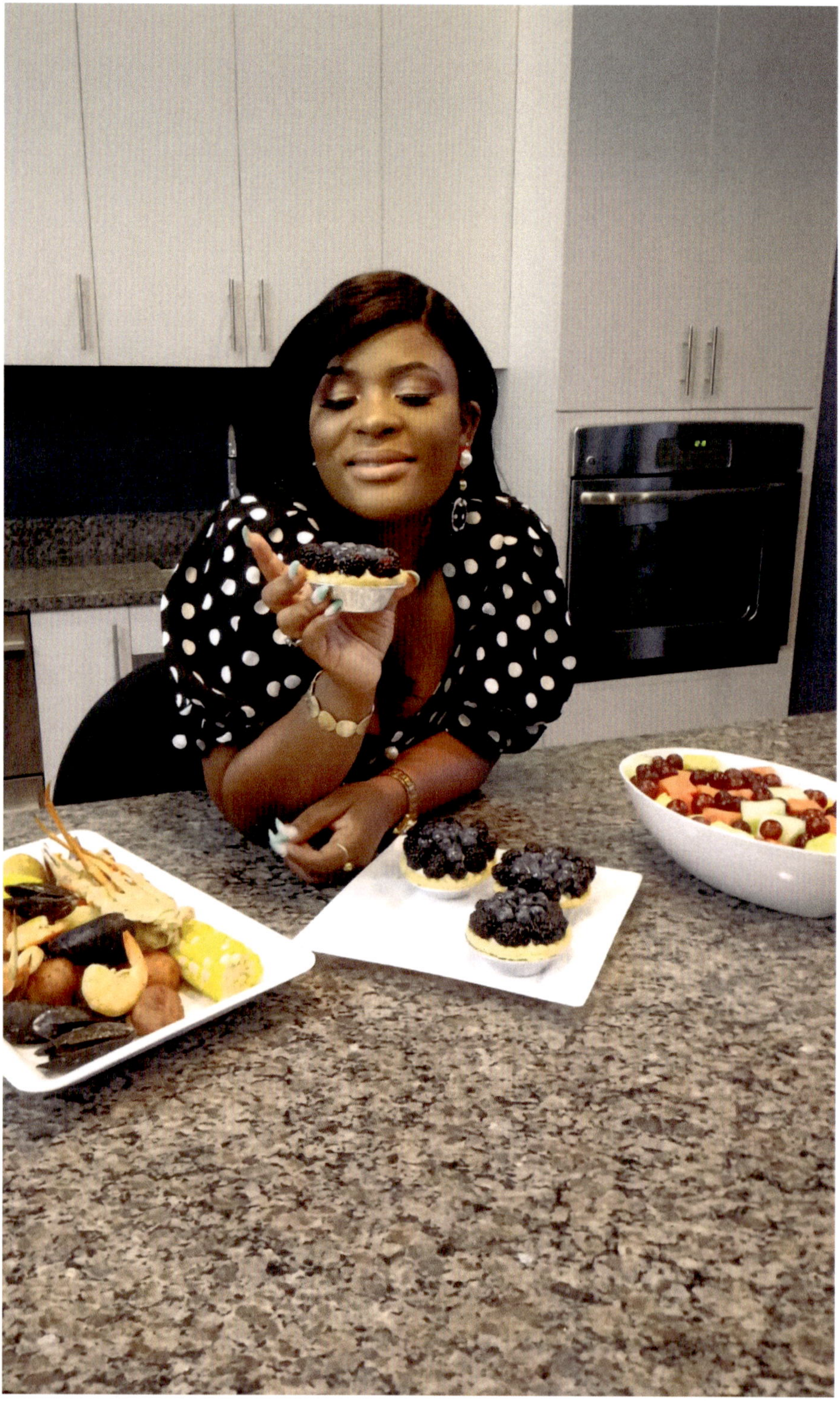

PREFACE

My name is Darline Dorcely, and I am the general manager of Chef Liline, a premium catering service based in Stamford, CT. I completed the hospitality management and culinary arts certification program at Norwalk Community College (NCC) in 2015. Additionally, I returned to school to earn an Associate of Science in Business Administration in 2019. Having a longstanding passion for cooking, I wanted to be able to apply my artistic talents to the culinary world. My passion and educational background led to specialized roles involving corporate teamwork, restaurants, hotels, country clubs, private parties, and large events.

I launched my business with a large tasting gathering and pleased the palettes of all my attendees. Today, I can be found all over social media, and on growing my YouTube channel where I am showcasing my skills to those who want to learn new recipes and be a mentor to other potential chefs in the near future. I am known best for my legendary service with a smile and best experiences ever!

I was born in Marchand Dessaline, Haiti, and spent most of my younger years there. Around 12 years old, I moved to the capital of Port-au-Prince, Haiti, and spent three years there until I came here to the United States. After my high school here in the US, I decided to pursue my interest in the culinary arts to learn more about cooking techniques, and it was the best decision I've ever made. When I was young, I was always watching my mother and other family members in the kitchen, putting love and care into every different type of dish they made. That sparked my passion for cooking every wonderful food, which is all about family, Sunday gathering, and celebrations. My family used to make griot is an absolute must-try traditional dish of Haiti; it was always my favorite. It is most often served with cabbage salad or, better yet, spicy pikliz. I remember one time I decided to cook my own; I asked mom to give me some uncooked pork meat, rice, and beans, so I could make my own food. I remember making griot and fried plantains, and we used to enjoy it. The food came so perfectly, and I kept on doing it every weekend. I always enjoyed cooking by adding my own flavor to it, and I could see the joy it brought into my family. Providing great meals for family members and friends is a happy moment for the Caribbean cooking, and each recipe within this book reflects that. Good times, good friends, and great food are what you want when you cook. And that's what this book will help you achieve! People love summertime because there are so many events happening, especially barbecue, which is natural for meals that are spur-of-the-moment gatherings, planned neighborhood feasts, or upscale patio dinner parties.

Caribbean food is not one dimensional; most people are unaware of how adaptable this type of cuisine really is. Many dishes combine very well with non-Caribbean dishes, while others are great on their own as snacks. These are just some of the reasons why Caribbean food is so popular in so many events.

What I love the most about Caribbean food is the taste of the stews, especially when you serve it on top of either cornmeal or rice; they are hearty, too. What makes Caribbean stews unique is the hint of warm sweet spices like clove and star anise.

My recipes are perfectly balanced between tradition, culture, and modern techniques. If you love exploring the foods of other cultures, then this cookbook is for you. I've compiled the very best recipes of the Caribbean into one beautiful layout, ready to adorn your kitchen shelf or coffee table. Just like the people, these dishes are diverse and influenced by various cultures. Caribbean dishes draw their inspiration from the many diverse cultures that make up the region.

The Caribbean has seen many visitors from different continents for centuries, most of whom have stayed back and formed grand lineages. One of the greatest cultural impacts of this migration has been on the food. The islands in the Caribbean have been fought over and owned by various European powers in the past, mainly the British, French, and Spanish. All of these cultures, as well as their respective culinary traditions, have played a role in forming the multinational cuisine of the Caribbean as it is nowadays.

Caribbean cuisine is a fusion of African, Amerindian, European, East Indian, Arab and Chinese cuisine. The indigenous population of the Caribbean added their own touch as well.

Caribbean food has a distinct flavor and a rich history. To decode its secrets, one must first give a respectful nod to the presence of its most vital ingredients: rice, plantains, beans, cassava, cilantro, bell peppers, chickpeas, tomatoes, sweet potatoes, and coconut, among others. This blend creates flavors as vibrant as the colors of the islands themselves. A peculiar seasoning tradition used in the region is based on green herbs and oil-based marinade. Ingredients may include garlic, onions, scotch bonnet peppers, celery, green onions, and herbs like cilantro, marjoram, rosemary, tarragon, and thyme. Used for many dishes, this marinade is one of the greatest secrets of Caribbean cuisine, and it is worth your time.

Food is an essential aspect of many family traditions and Caribbean culture. People from countries like Haiti, Dominican Republic, Bahamas, Jamaica, and Trinidad, just to mention a few, spend considerably longer times cooking than going to a restaurant to buy food. We enjoy being in the kitchen because it's like a therapy for us. We usually dance while we are cooking; that's why the food always comes so perfect and tasty.

A LITTLE TIP BEFORE COOKING

Give yourself some time to get the best that you can afford and, when possible, choose the best organic ingredients to create tasty Caribbean food. Enjoy every minute to become your best friend in the kitchen and the main cheerleader for your future tasty yummy food.

KITCHEN MEASUREMENT CONVERSION TABLES

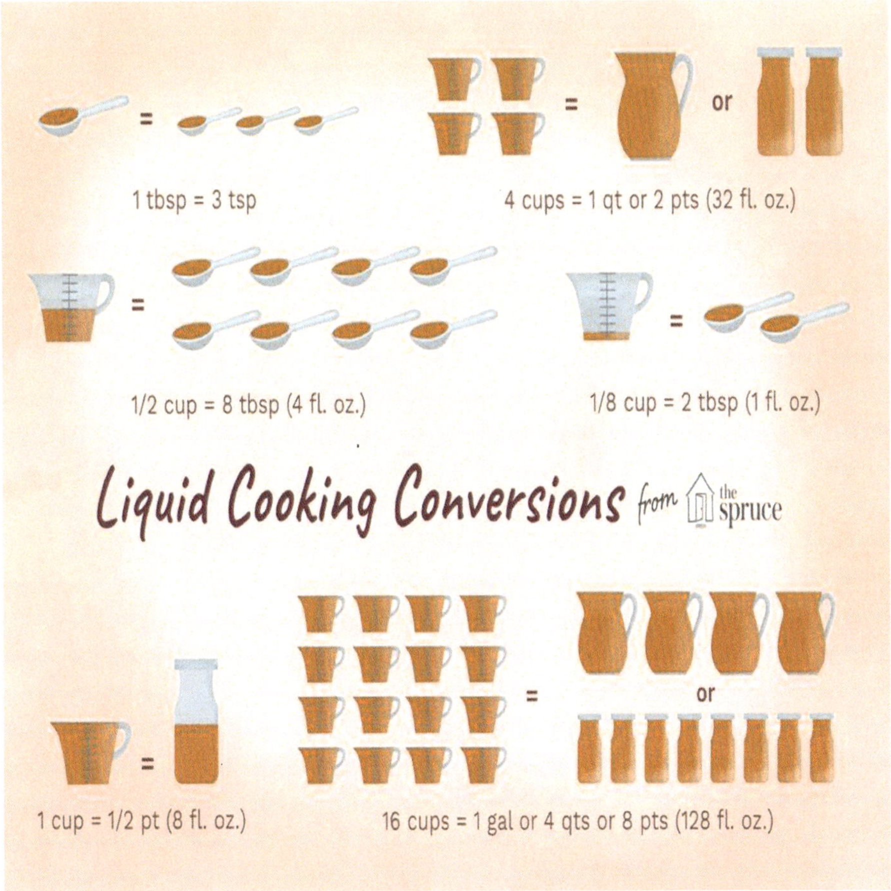

01 APPETIZERS

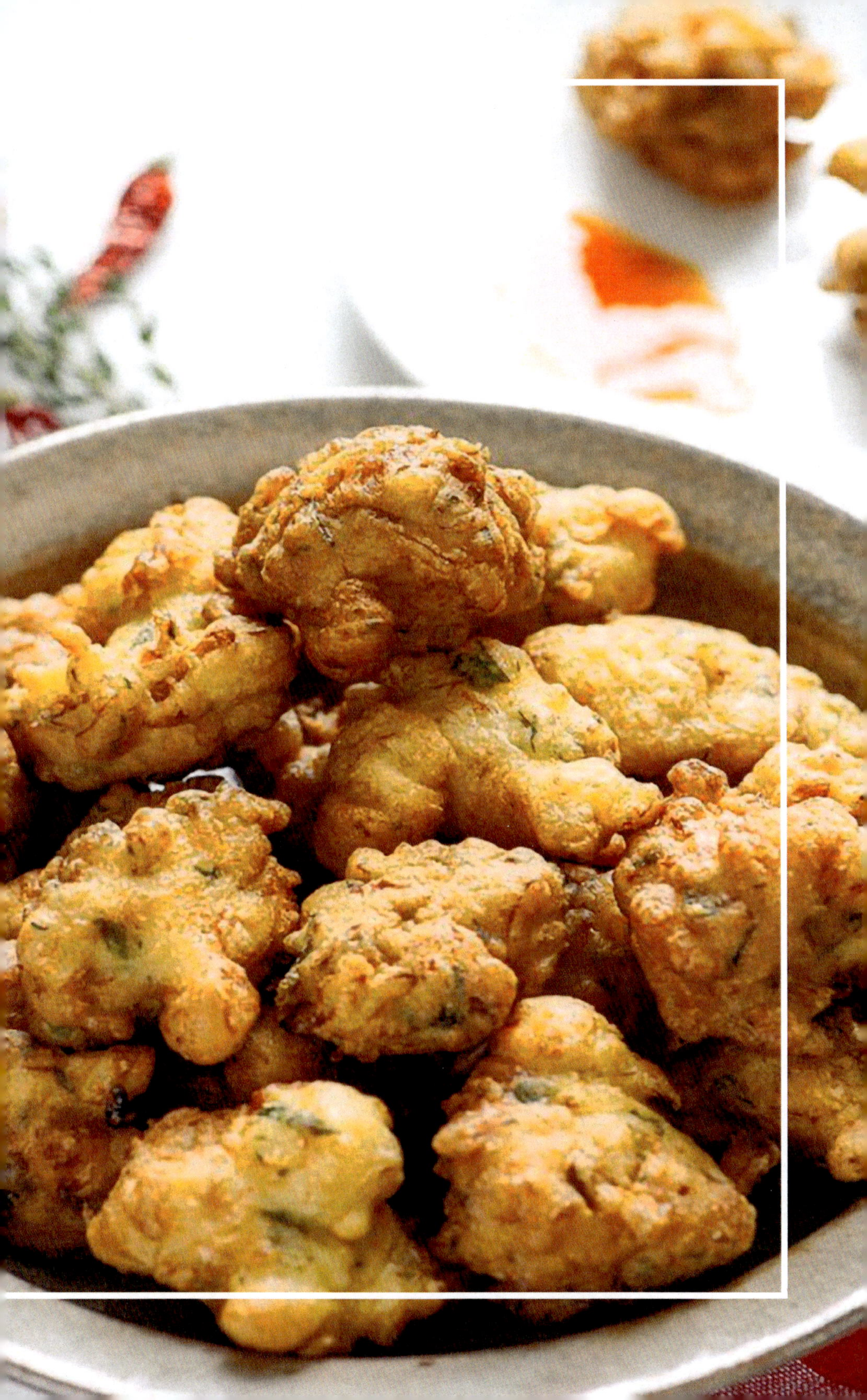

POTATO-CODFISH CROQUETTES

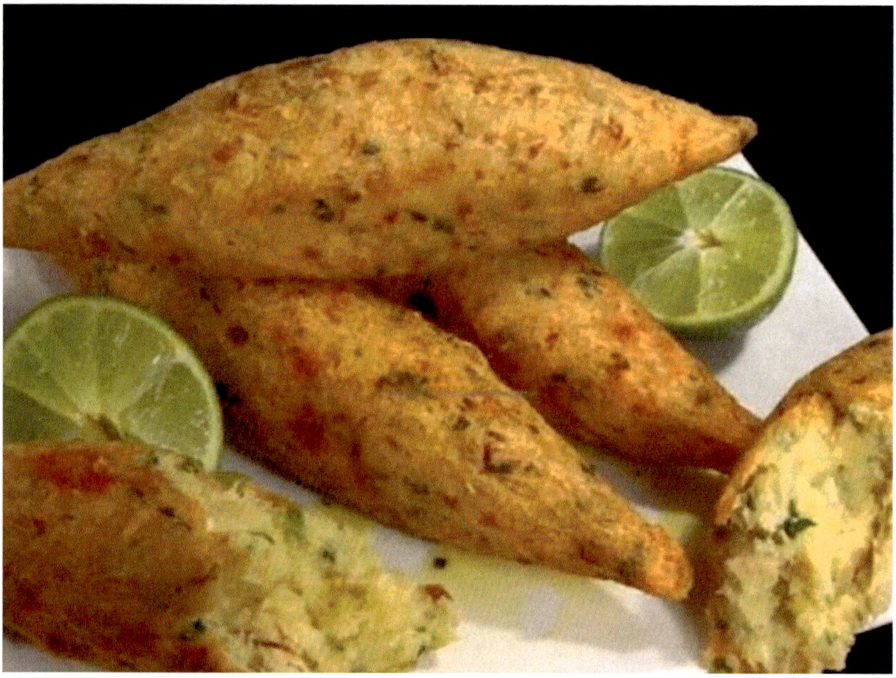

INGREDIENTS

- 4 potatoes
- 1 lb of salted cod fish pieces (morue, bacalao)
- Parsley and thyme
- Scotch bonnet peppers (you can also use red pepper flakes)
- Salt (if needed), black pepper
- Garlic
- 3 radishes
- 2 tbsps of butter
- 1 onion

INSTRUCTIONS

1. The procedure to desalt the cod fish is the same as the one for unsalting smoked herring.
2. Fill a recipient of water at room temperature. Leave your cod fish soak inside the bowl for 10 to 12 hours or simply overnight. Change the water as often as you think you should. Check for saltiness.
3. Clean your fish with white vinegar and massage it with two lemon halves. Drain out the lemon. Leave just a little bit to boil with the water.
4. Fill a pot with water. Not too much. Just enough to cover the fish. Let it boil for 10-15 mins.
5. Once you're done boiling, drain the water out and start" fishing" for bones. Take out the very hard bones.
6. Tear the fish into small little pieces. That part should be easy because this will tend to happen as you're taking out the bones. I used a fork and a knife to do so, but you may do it your own way.
7. Boil your potatoes until very tender. Peel off the skin.
8. Cut your onions and radishes into dice. Add garlic, black pepper, salt (if you think your fish doesn't have enough salt), thyme, parsley, and crushed Caribbean pepper. BLEND! This will allow for the flavors to be well mixed with the potato and fish.
9. Grab a big bowl and add onion mix, fish, and potato into it. Now using your hands, massage them all together (if you think you might need gloves, don't hesitate to use them)
10. Add your 2 tbsps of butter and massage again.
11. Grease a cookie sheet. Separate your mix into small little balls and bake at 350F
12. It should be ready in 20 to 30 mins. The more gold it gets, the more you can think it's ready.
13. (If you prefer to fry these, form the mix into boo balls. Roll in seasoned flour to coat. Then fry until golden brown.)

SHRIMP AVOCADO PLANTAINS CUPS

If there's one food I can't live without, it's plantains. Green, ripe, sweet or starchy, boiled, fried, mashed, They're so versatile and are definitely more satisfying than a plain old potato. If you're looking for ways to switch up those boring carbs on your plate, plantains are the way to go! My favorite thing to do with plantains is making fried plantain cups! Bread bowls, move aside! This tostones rellenos is an awesome hand-held appetizer or dinner option that will truly impress your guests.

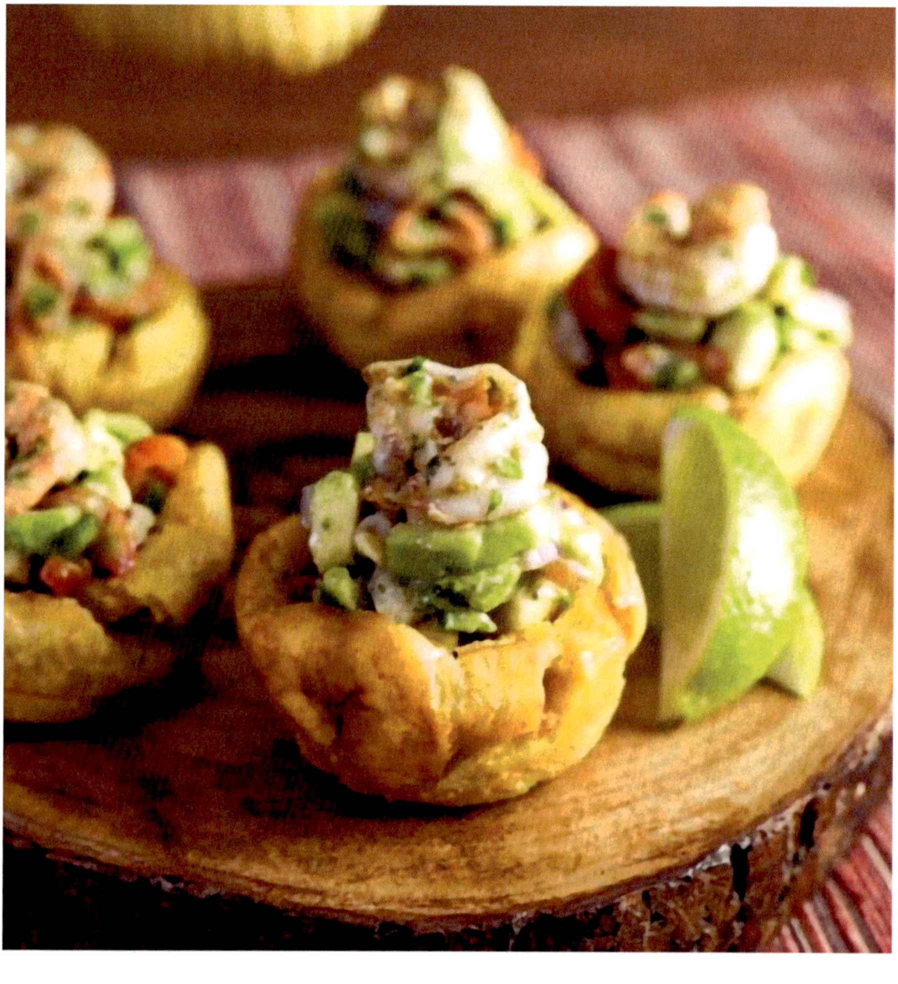

INGREDIENTS

Seafood

12 Shrimps

Produce

1 Avocado, ripe

1/4 cup of Cherry tomatoes

1 tbsp of Cilantro

1 Garlic clove

1 Jalapeno, small

2 Plantains, green

1/4 cup of red onion

Condiments

3 tbsp of Lime juice

Baking & Spices

1 Salt and pepper

Oils & kinds of vinegar

1 Vegetable or canola oil

Nuts & Seeds

1/2 tsp of Cumin powder

INSTRUCTIONS

1. Season shrimps with salt, pepper, and cumin powder. Cook in a lightly oiled skillet. Then place in a bowl, along with the avocado, tomatoes, jalapeño, garlic, red onion, cilantro, and lime juice. Mix well and chill in the fridge.
2. Peel and slice plantains into 3-inch chunks. Fry in 350F oil until slightly golden, but not browned, for about 4-5 minutes.
3. Immediately place one fried plantain chunk each in a greased muffin pan well. Using a pestle or shot glass, gently press to form a cup.
4. Fry again until golden brown. Drain on a paper towel and lightly season with salt.
5. Immediately fill the cups with the shrimp mixture and serve.

KIBBEH

Making a great kibbe is an art form and can take a lot of practice to get just right. You have to make sure the kibbe is crunchy but not too dry. The casing has to be thin but still substantial enough to balance the filling. The filling should complement the casing without overwhelming it. When you bite a kibbe, it should be savory and moderately spiced, never too spicy or bland. So many things to consider but not impossible to perfect. This recipe is for individually fried morsels, but can also be adapted to the kibbeh, which is baked.

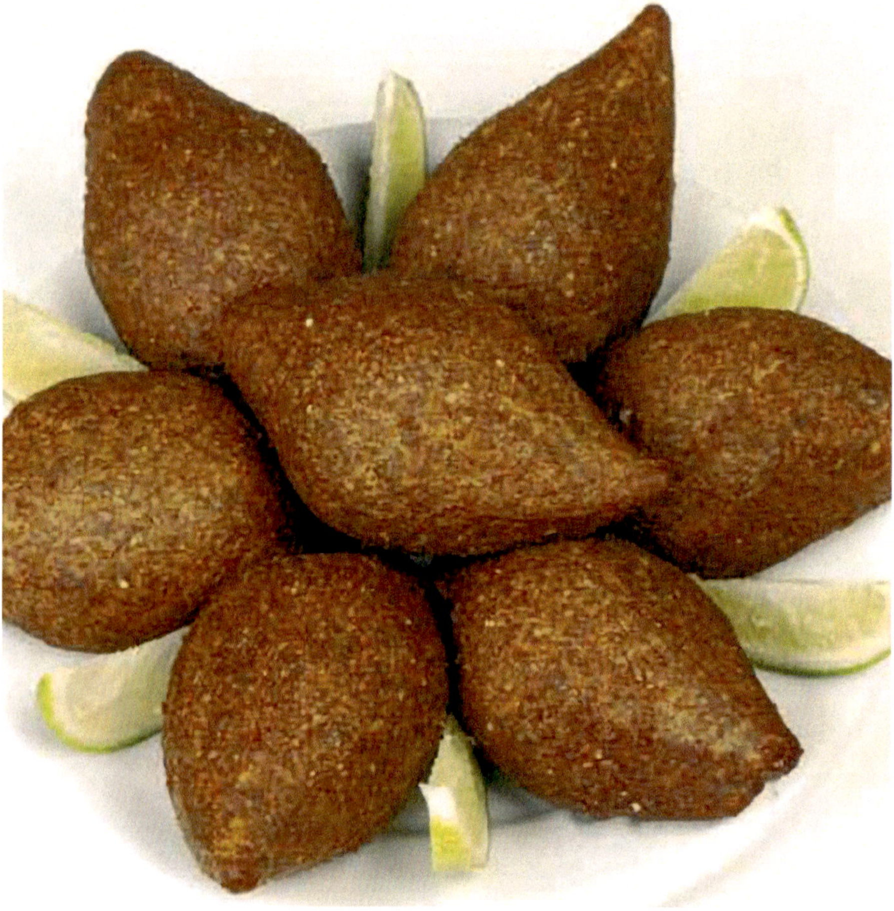

INGREDIENTS

1 tsp of allspice	1 tsp of salt
1/4 tsp of cumin	1 tsp of pepper
2 tbsps of olive oil	1 tsp of salt for the filling
2 garlic cloves, crushed and minced	1tsp of pepper for the filling
2 medium onions (1 coarsely chopped and the other one finely minced)	1/2 lb. (1 cup) of Bulgar cracked wheat (make sure it's finely crushed and not coarse)
5 dried or smoked herring fillet, cut in small pieces or 2 lbs finely ground beef	slices of lemon

INSTRUCTIONS

1. Soak the Bulgar wheat in cold water for 1/2 hour minimum
2. Remove your Bulgar wheat from water. Dry by removing excess water. Then add to the 1 lb of meat, coarsely chopped onions, pepper, and salt.
3. KIBBEH STUFFING PREPARATION In a medium frying pan, saute the finely chopped onion in olive oil. Add ground beef and chop well with a wooden spoon. Add allspice, salt, pepper, and cumin. Once the beef is light brown, remove from heat. Allow it to cool for 10 minutes. (You're also allowed to add any other ingredients of your will. I personally thought that it needed some more. Be Haitian, Be bold, and allow your taste buds to be part of the decision making)
4. Take an egg-sized amount of shell mixture and form it into a ball. With your finger, poke a hole in the ball, making space for filling. Add filling and pinch the top to seal the ball. You can then shape it into a point, or football shape, or leave as a ball.
5. Fry in 350-degree oil on a stove top or in a deep fryer for about 10 minutes or until golden brown. Drain on paper towels.
6. Serve with slices of lemon.

CONCH FRITTERS WITH CARIBBEAN DIPPING SAUCE

A spiced batter littered with fresh conch meat is deep-fried until golden. These conch fritters are a little taste of the islands that are downright addicting! I think one of the best ways to see the Caribbean is to cruise the Caribbean! There is so much to love about cruising, but one of the best things is to be able to tour several different islands or countries in one trip.

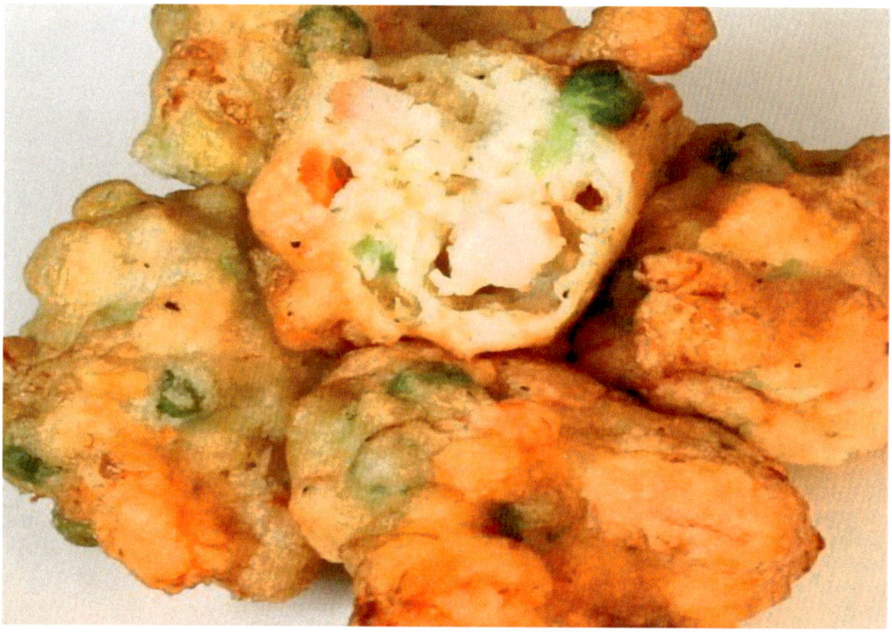

INGREDIENTS

Fritters:

1 cup of all-purpose flour

3 teaspoons of baking powder

sea salt and fresh-ground black pepper to taste

INSTRUCTIONS

Fritters:

1. In a large mixing bowl, whisk together the flour, baking powder, salt, and pepper.
2. In another bowl, combine the ground conch, green and red peppers, onions, and garlic,

1 cup of firm-packed ground conch or shrimp

1/2 green bell pepper, finely chopped

1/2 red bell pepper, finely chopped

1 small onion, finely chopped

2 medium garlic cloves, minced

1/2 cup of milk

1 large egg

1 teaspoon of fresh lime juice

dash Tabasco to taste

canola oil for frying

Caribbean Dipping Sauce:

1/2 cup of prepared salsa

1 cup of real mayonnaise

1 teaspoon of garlic powder

1/4 teaspoon of cayenne pepper

1/2 teaspoon of dried basil, crushed

1/2 teaspoon of salt, plus more to taste

1/4 teaspoon of fresh-ground black pepper

making sure the conch is well distributed. Add the conch mixture to the flour mixture.

3. Without cleaning the conch bowl, use it to whisk together the milk, egg, lime juice, and Tabasco. Add to the conch mixture, stirring until everything is well mixed. Cover and refrigerate up to an hour so the batter firms a bit.
4. When ready to finish, heat about 1/4-inch oil in a large, heavy skillet over medium-high heat. Place about a heaping tablespoon of conch batter for each fritter carefully into the skillet, without crowding. This may have to be done in batches. Press down very lightly on each portion of batter to flatten. The fritters will spread slightly.
5. Cook 1 1/2 to 2 minutes per side or until nicely browned and cooked through. Transfer to paper towels to drain. You may want to keep the fritters warm in a 200°F oven while you cook all the batter to keep them warm, but this is optional.
6. To serve, place six fritters on each of four warm dishes. Place about six tablespoons of dipping sauce in four small bowls. Serve one with each serving.

Caribbean Dipping Sauce:

1. In a blender, puree the salsa—place in a nonreactive bowl. Add the remaining ingredients and whisk well. Cover and refrigerate for several hours. Stir before serving. Makes about 1 1/2 cups.

JAMAICAN SALT FISH FRITTERS

Jamaican Salt fish fritter is simply delicious. Well flavored with scallion, thyme, onion, scotch bonnet pepper mix with salt fish and flour. All these ingredients fuse together to give you that great taste of the Jamaican salt fish fritter that you are going to try today. The selling point for salt fish fritter is the scotch bonnet pepper, at least for me, I love spicy food. The scotch bonnet pepper should be just enough, so you know that it is in the fritters but not too much that you have to drink water while eating the fritters.

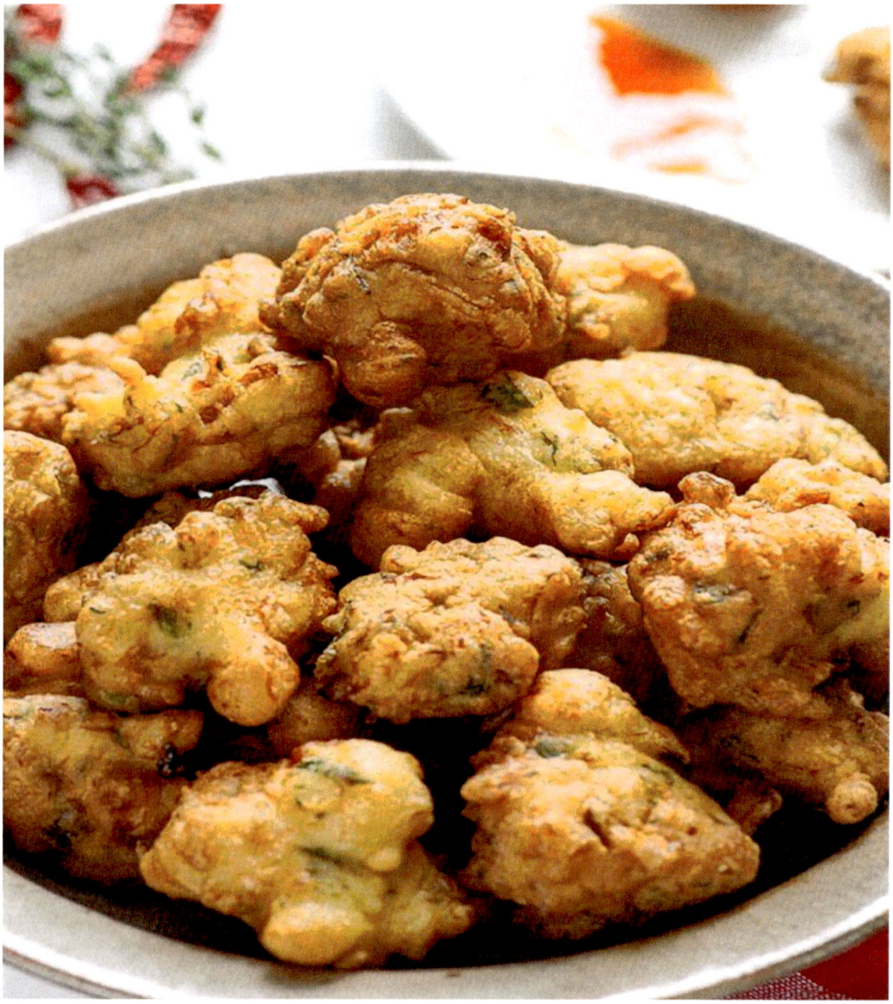

INGREDIENTS

2 tbsp of Bell pepper

1 tsp of Garlic, granulated

1/2 of Onion, medium

3 tbsp of Parsley

1/2 tsp of Scotch bonnet pepper

1 tsp of Thyme, fresh

1 Egg, large

Baking & Spices

1 cup of All-purpose flour

2 tsp of Baking powder

1/2 tsp of Paprika, smoked

1 Pepper

1/2 tsp of Sugar

Oils & Vinegar

1 Vegetable oil

Liquids

1/3 cup of milk or water

Other

1/2 pound of boneless salted cod fish, or use any white fish

INSTRUCTIONS

1. Soak salt fish in water overnight or several days (water changed several times). Drain and shred fish using a food processor to achieve a really fine shred. If not finely shred by hands
2. Combine the dry ingredients, flour baking powder, smoked paprika, granulated garlic, and sugar. Stir for about a minute then add onions, salted shredded fish, thyme, and red bell pepper, scotch bonnet parsley, and egg
3. Whisk until ingredients have been blended. Then add milk gradually starting from about 1/3 cup until the desired thickness.
4. Adjust seasonings.
5. You may have to do a test taste first
6. Heat oil to 350 degrees in a skillet or saucepan. You may also use the oil test by dropping a 1-inch square of bread into the oil. If it takes 60 seconds to brown, then the oil is at around 350 degrees.
7. Carefully place spoonfuls of the batter into the hot oil and fry for 3-4- minutes or until the fritters are crisp and golden-brown (you may need to do this in batches). Remove from the pan with a slotted spoon and set aside.
8. You may drain on a paper napkin to remove any excess oil

THE BEST HOMEMADE DINNER ROLLS

The Best Homemade Dinner Rolls are buttery, fluffy, and taste heavenly! These homemade rolls will be gone in no time in your home. It is side dish week on Modern Honey, so I can't wait to share everything I have been whipping up in my kitchen. These best Homemade Dinner Rolls are heaven-sent. These rolls are made with simple ingredients: yeast, water, sugar, butter, milk, flour, and salt. It's the ratios that matter. The dough has just the right amount of butter to make them melt-in-your-mouth, rolls and enough yeast to help them rise and make them fluffy. Buttery, light, fluffy homemade dinner rolls are a must in our home! I am sharing all of the tips and tricks to make perfect dinner rolls every single time.

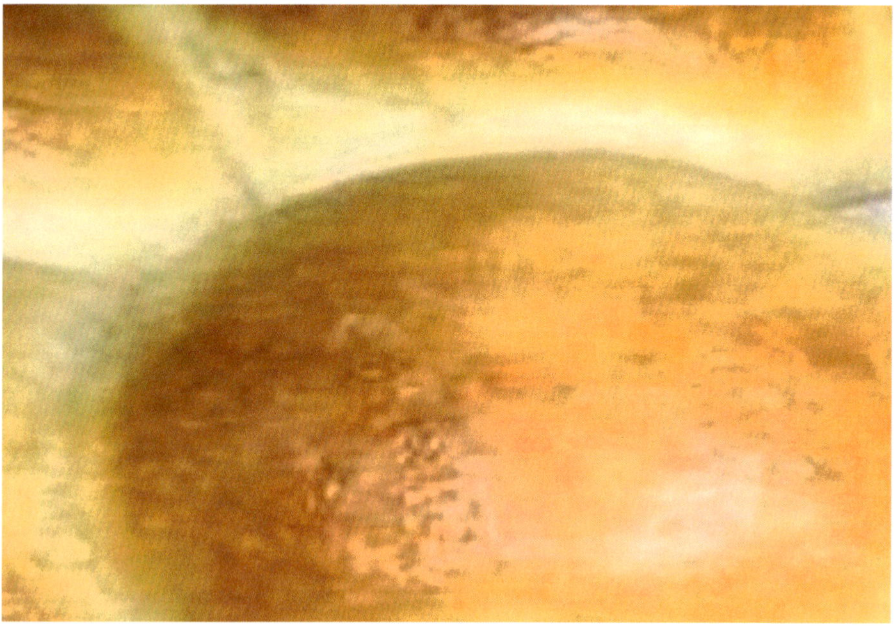

INGREDIENTS

1/2 cup of canned pineapple juice (room temperature)

1/2 cup of warm milk (100 – 110°F)

4 tablespoons of unsalted butter, melted and slightly cooled

2 whole eggs, lightly beaten

6 tablespoons of granulated sugar

1 1/2 teaspoons of fine salt

2 1/4 teaspoons (1 packet) of instant yeast

4 1/2 cups (20 ounces) of bread flour

Combine the pineapple juice, milk, melted butter, eggs, sugar, salt, and yeast in the bowl of a stand mixer. Add 2 cups of the flour and stir with a wooden spoon until the dough forms a rough, shaggy mass. Attach the dough hook to the mixer and turn to medium-low speed. Gradually add the remaining flour JUST until the dough comes together. You may not need all the flour, depending on your kitchen environment and brand of flour. Continue kneading at medium-high speed for 4 to 5 minutes, until a soft and smooth ball of dough forms.

INSTRUCTIONS

1. Place the dough in a clean bowl. Cover with plastic wrap. Leave to rise until puffy and doubled in size, about 1 hour.
2. Spray a 13x9-inch baking pan with cooking spray. Gently deflate the dough. Use a bench scraper or knife to divide the dough into 15 equal pieces. Shape each piece into a ball and place it in the prepared pan.
3. In a small bowl, combine the egg with two tablespoons of water. Brush all over the rolls. Cover with plastic wrap and let rise again until doubled in size, about 30 minutes.
4. Meanwhile, preheat the oven to 375°F.
5. Bake the rolls for 20 minutes, or until golden brown. Serve warm.

STUFFED BAKED SWEET PLANTAINS

Similar to a Puerto Rico Pastelon, which is really more of a plantain lasagna. Instead, these are made as individual boats that are easy to make, filling, and perfect as a main dish.

If you're not very familiar with plantains, they are similar to bananas, only that they need to be cooked. Green plantains are usually meant for salty chips or tostones, but when the plantains are very ripe, almost black, that's when they are at their sweetest! That's what you want here, not yellow because they won't be sweet and soft enough. They should be soft, and the skin almost black.

INGREDIENTS

Meat

1/2 lb. Ground meat

Produce

1 tsp of Garlic

1/2 Onion, medium

2 tbsp of Parsley

2 Plantains, ripe

Condiments

1/2 cup of Tomato sauce

Baking & Spices

1 tbsp of Paprika, smoked

1 Salt and pepper

1 Yellow or red pepper, small green

Oils & Vinegars

2 tbsp of Canola oil

1 Cooking spray

Dairy

1/2 cup of cheese, grated

INSTRUCTIONS

1. Preheat the oven to 400°F. Line baking sheets with foil and coat with cooking spray or oil.
2. Using a sharp knife, cut both ends off the plantain. This will make it easy to grab the skin of the plantains. Slit a shallow line down the long seam of the plantain, peel only as deep as the peel. Remove plantain peel by pulling back.
3. Place plantains on a tray and lightly spray, bake for about 15, turn and bake on the other side for another 15 minutes or until golden brown and tender.
4. While the plantains are baking, add 2 tablespoons of oil to a saucepan, followed by onions, garlic, and tomato sauce. Let it simmer for about 10 minutes, frequently stirring to prevent burning, add about ½ cup of water if needed.
5. Then, add ground meat and continue cooking for about 10 or more minutes.
6. Finally, add green pepper and parsley, adjust for seasoning
7. Remove baked plantains from oven cool for a couple of minutes, make a horizontal slit in the plantains, stuff with equal amounts of the meat mixture
8. Sprinkle with cheese, if desired, place in the oven and bake for an additional 5 minutes. Serve warm

CARIBBEAN GREEN LIVING

One of my absolute favorite Haitian foods is Accra. It's generally made with ground black eye peas and/or grated malanga, seasoned with spices (let's not forget the scotch bonnet) and fried.

Brazil has a similar dish called acarajé, which is split in half once fried and stuffed with shrimp, ground cashews, etc. The native version of both is called Akara and seems to have originated from western Africa.

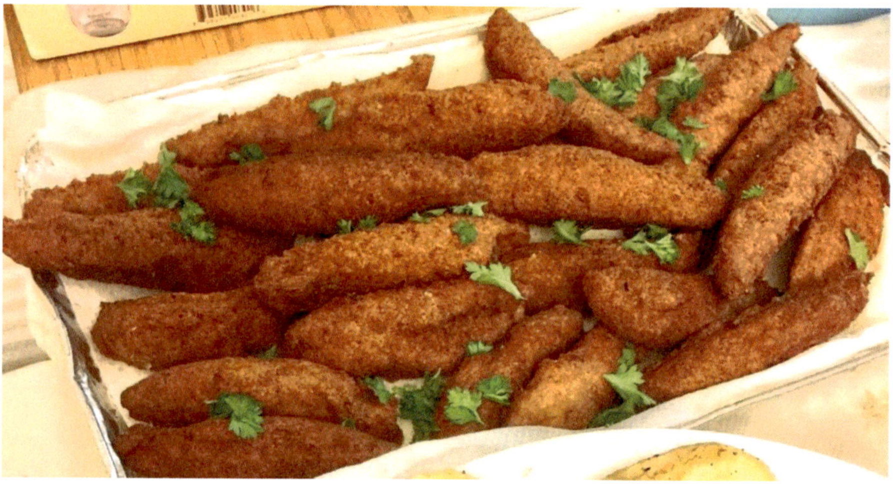

INGREDIENTS

1 lb. malanga cut into 2.5cm (1" pieces)

2 scallions chopped

2 cloves of garlic

2 tablespoons of parsley chopped

1 teaspoon of thyme leaves only

2 tablespoons of green peppers chopped

campaign icon Coupons

¼ teaspoon of ground black pepper

1 teaspoon of salt plus more to taste

½ tablespoon of scotch bonnet pepper or Habanero, chopped seeds and membrane removed

1 – 2 tablespoons of all-purpose flour

1 tablespoon of olive oil, if baking

2 cups of vegetable oil if frying only

INSTRUCTIONS

1. Peel all Malangas and cut pieces into smaller 2.5cm (1") cubes.
2. Add to the food processor.
3. Add all ingredients also to the food processor with the exception of oils.
4. Blend all ingredients to a smooth mixture, including olive oil, if BAKING ONLY.
5. Put the mixture in a bowl, cover, and let marinate in the refrigerator for 30 minutes or longer.
6. Blend all ingredients into a smooth mixture.
7. Remove and add to a bowl without olive oil if FRYING ONLY.
8. Cover and let marinate in the refrigerator for 30 minutes or longer.
9. Remove mixture from the refrigerator and let it stand at room temperature. If frying, mix with flour and with 2 dinner spoons, shape the accra and fry golden brown in hot oil. Serve hot.
10. If baking – When ready, butter 2 – 3 ramekins.
11. Fill ramekins with Accra mixture, do with butter and bake at 190°C / 375°F / Gas Mark 5 for 30 to 35 minutes.
12. You may change the temperature of the oven to broil for the top to crisp, but no more than 5 minutes. Serve hot.

PLANTAIN BURGER

If you've ever tried Cuban-style tostones (aka fried plantains), then you'll love this recipe! Combining only three ingredients, this dish is completely gluten-free and easy to make. It's subtle sweet flavor compliments savory burger patties with a tropical twist. The best part is, you don't even need to turn on the oven. Plantains are naturally starchy and hold up exceptionally well when pan-frying or baking. Similar to bananas, they're high in potassium and fiber, while packing in plenty of probiotics. Peak ripeness occurs when their yellow peels have brown or black marks, but even a black plantain is fully acceptable here. The peel of a plantain is usually tough and sometimes requires scoring with a sharp knife to remove. On the inside, the flesh should be firm and ready for mashing into "buns" without needing to add in any eggs. Arrowroot powder helps absorb some of the plantain's moisture. It adds a crispy texture to the buns while adding enough elasticity to pile on the toppings. Use it to thicken the mashed plantains and to withstand high-temperature cooking. If you don't have any on hand, use tapioca starch or cassava flour instead.

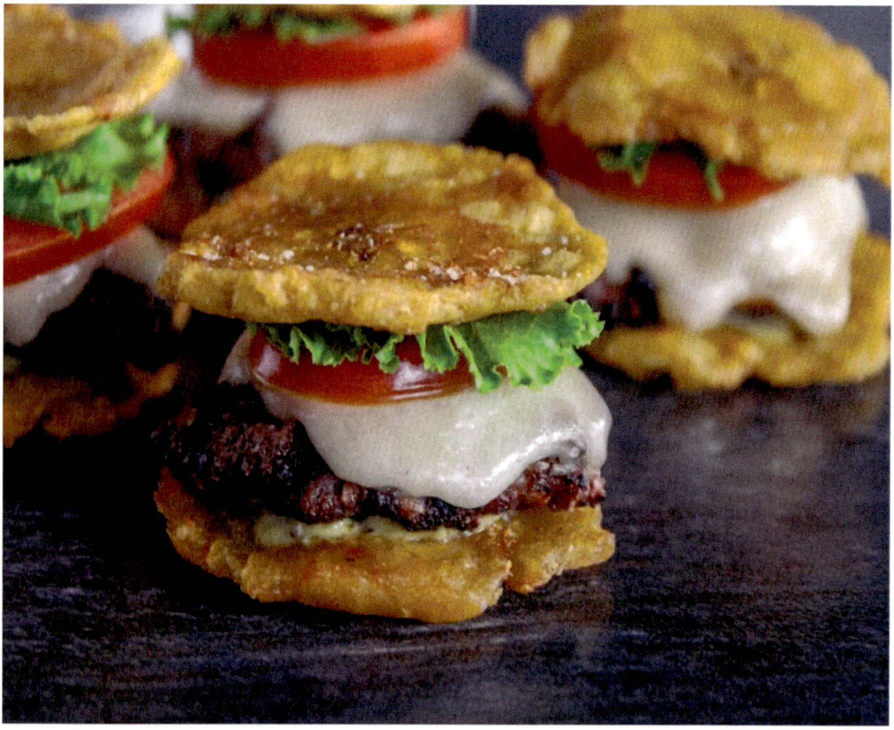

INGREDIENTS

2 Plantains (ripe & firm)

2 Burger Patties

1 Fresh Beef Tomato (sliced)

1 Onion (Sliced)

¼ Bunch of Lettuce

2-4 Cheese Slices

Olive Oil

4 Tablespoons of Ketchup

4 Tablespoons of Mayonnaise

½ Slice of Lemon

Salt and Pepper (to taste)

Spices (to taste)

INSTRUCTIONS

1. Spice the burger patties with salt, pepper, and spices. Place them in the grill or pre-oiled heated pan and allow them to cook until your preferred level of 'cooked' is reached. Be sure to flip the patties over at intervals
2. Whilst the patties are still piping hot, place the slices of cheese on them to melt
3. For the plantains, wash, peel and cut each one into two and place in a pan of heated olive oil. Allow them to cook slightly, then remove from the pan and mash into a thick paste. You can add some salt at this point
4. Use a roller (or anything that works like a roller) to flatten the mashed paste to about ½ inch, then place it in the heated pan a second time until cooked. Remember to flip them over at intervals while they cook
5. Place the fried plantains on paper towels to absorb any excess oil
6. Now, assemble the burger patties (with melted cheese), sliced tomatoes and onions, and plantains in the typical burger arrangement. Plantain -> patty (with melted cheese) -> tomatoes, onions, lettuce -> plantain.
7. Serve with pink sauce (mix the ketchup, mayonnaise, and a few drops of lemon. Stir until pink and thoroughly combined).

FRIED PLANTAINS WITH AVOCADO AND GRILLED SHRIMP

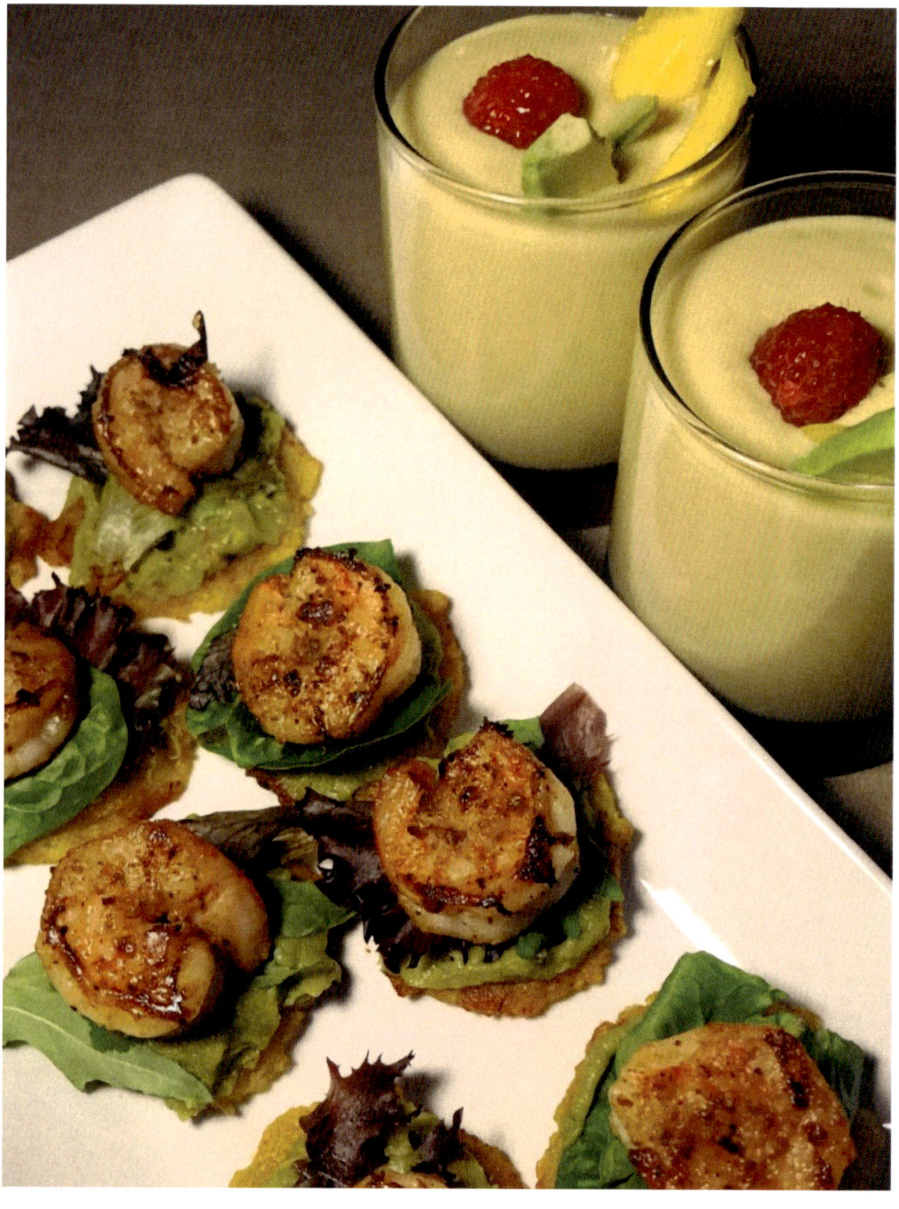

INGREDIENTS

- 4 plantains
- 1 cup of oil for frying
- 2 tablespoons of olive oil
- 4 cloves of garlic crushed into a paste
- 20 jumbo shrimp, peeled
- 1 teaspoon of salt (or more, to taste)
- 1 large avocado
- Juice of 1 lime
- 1/4 teaspoon of pepper (or more, to taste)

INSTRUCTIONS

To make the cups

1. Preheat the oven to 200 F [100 ºC].
2. Peel the bananas (or plantains). Cut into 6 slices each banana or 7 slices each plantain. Heat oil for frying over medium temperature.
3. Fry each slice until they are golden brown all over. Squeeze the slices using a lemon squeezer forming small cups. Once all the cups are formed, fry them again over medium heat until all the light parts have turned golden brown.
4. Turn off the oven and leave the cups in the oven while you go-ahead to the next step.

For the shrimp

1. Heat the olive oil over very low heat. Add the garlic and shallots. I also seasoned with liline creole seafood seasoning for a better taste and let it cook for 3 to 4 minutes. Do not let the garlic burn. Add the shrimp and cook until they are pink throughout. Season with salt to taste and pepper.
2. Remove from the heat and reserve.

For the avocado

5. Peel avocado and crush using a fork until it doesn't have any lumps. Mix in the lime juice.
6. Season with salt and pepper to taste.
7. To assemble
8. Spoon about a tablespoon of avocado mix into the cups.
9. Top each with a shrimp and garnish with cilantro leaves.
10. Serve immediately.

Tips and Notes

If you use plantains, skip the oven step, as plantains get dry and hard too easily.

FRIED PLANTAINS

Today we're talking about plantains, which are a member of the banana family, but they are lower in sugar. Plantains are common in the Caribbean and are often eaten more like a vegetable than a fruit.

Fried plantains are just what they sound like, plantains that have been fried! Plantains look similar to bananas, but they don't have the same flavor. As plantains fry, the edges become crispy and slightly caramelized with just barely a sweet touch of flavor. They are great eaten as a snack or as an appetizer.

You can actually fry plantains in just about any stage of ripeness. When making twice-fried plantains (or tostones), you'll want to use a green plantain. They are great for making plantain chips at this point.

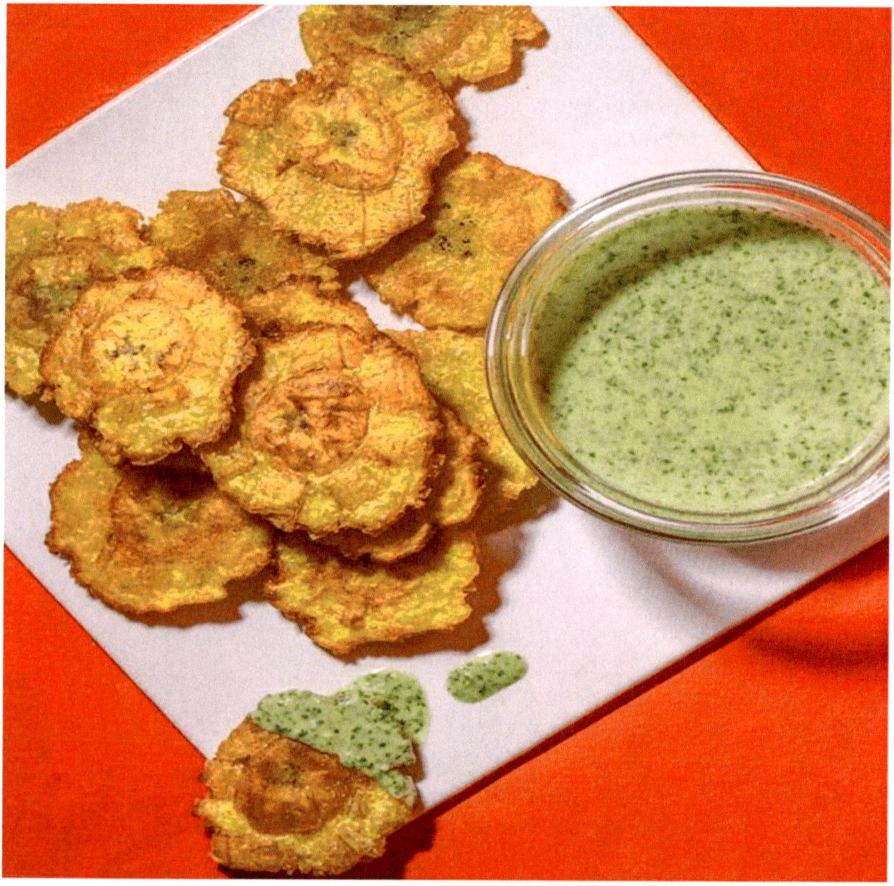

INGREDIENTS

2 large green plantains

¼ cup of coconut oil, divided

1-2 tsp of garlic salt (depending on how salty you like them!)

INSTRUCTIONS

1. Set up your workstation: a large cutting board next to the stove, a medium-sized skillet, a wooden spatula for smashing the plantains, and a small cookie sheet (or plate) prepared by sprinkling garlic salt all over it.
2. Prepare the plantains for frying: cut off each end, then make a slit down the length of the entire plantain and peel back the skin. You may need to use a knife to remove any remaining parts of the skin still on the plantain.
3. Cut the plantains into ½ - ¾ inch slices.
4. Heat a medium-sized skillet with 2 Tbsp of coconut oil over medium heat for 2 minutes to allow the oil to get hot.
5. Once the oil is ready, carefully slide the plantains down the side of the skillet, so you don't splash yourself with oil.
6. Cook the plantains for 2 minutes on the first side, until golden brown. Use a fork to turn each plantain over. I like to use the side of the pan to help me flip them. Cook an additional 2 minutes on the second side.
7. Remove the plantains to a cutting board or plate on the side, add an additional 2 Tbsp oil to the pan, then turn OFF the heat.
8. Use the back of a wooden spatula (or bottom of a glass jar) to flatten the plantains until they're about ¼ inch thick.
9. Turn the heat back on the pan, and add an additional 2 Tbsp of coconut oil.
10. Slide the plantains back in, and cook for about a minute to a 1 minute 30 seconds on both sides, until they're even more golden brown and delicious. You may need to do this in two batches depending on the size of your pan.
11. Once they're finished cooking, remove the plantains immediately to the cookie sheet and toss the tostones with garlic salt.
12. Eat up!

CARIBBEAN STYLE CORN ON THE COB

The way you eat corn on the cob will never be the same after you've tried this mouthwatering Caribbean-style recipe.

INGREDIENTS

- 6 ears of fresh corn or sweet corn
- 1 large egg yolk
- 1 teaspoon of Dijon mustard
- 3/4 cup of extra virgin olive oil
- 1 clove of garlic
- 1 teaspoon of sea salt
- 1/2 teaspoon of ground black pepper
- 1 tablespoon of lemon juice
- 3 tablespoons of fresh parsley, finely chopped, divided
- Paprika and grated Parmesan cheese for serving

INSTRUCTIONS

1. Preheat the oven to 350°F.
2. Make a cut around the bright green husks of the corn at 2 inches from the end. Tear off the husks along with the cut. (See photos. This step is to turn the corn cob into a handle.) Remove the silk inside.
3. Wrap up each prepared ear of corn with aluminum foil and put directly on the oven rack. Bake for 30-35 minutes.
4. While the corn is baking, make the aioli. Smash up the garlic with sea salt with a pestle and mortar (or use the end of a rolling pin in a metal bowl).
5. Place egg yolk and mustard in a medium bowl. Whisk until blended. Start adding oil, bit by bit, stirring vigorously till creamy. Make sure to blend well each time you add a bit of oil into the egg yolk mixture.
6. When all the oil has gone in, and the mixture is thickened, add lemon juice and the smashed garlic with salt. Mix well. Add two tablespoons of chopped parsley. Stir until evenly mixed. Taste, season with more salt, pepper, or lemon juice if needed.
7. When corn is done, let cool for a few minutes.
8. Coat each ear of corn with two tablespoons of aioli. Make sure that all sides are covered. Sprinkle it with paprika and Parmesan cheese. To finish off, top with the remaining parsley.

TURKEY PICADILLO

INGREDIENTS

6 medium ripe plantains, peeled

12 tbsp of shredded part-skim mozzarella cheese

fresh cilantro, for garnish

For the Turkey Picadillo:

10 oz 93% lean ground turkey

1/4 cup of onion, finely chopped

2 cloves of minced garlic

1/2 medium tomato, chopped

1/4 cup of bell pepper, finely chopped

2 tbsp of cilantro

2 oz tomato sauce

kosher salt

fresh ground pepper

3/4 tsp of ground cumin

1/8 tsp of oregano

1 bay leaf

1 tbsp of alcaparrado, capers, or green olives would work too

INSTRUCTIONS

1. Preheat the oven to 400°F.
2. Cut a split lengthwise through the length of the plantain about halfway through. Place them on a baking dish and bake covered with foil until soft, about 40 minutes.
3. Meanwhile, brown the ground turkey on medium heat in a large sauté pan and season with salt and pepper. Use a wooden spoon to break the meat up into small pieces.
4. Add the chopped onions, garlic, pepper, tomato, and cilantro and continue cooking on low heat.
5. Add alcaparrado (or olives and capers) and about 2 tbsp of the brine (this adds great flavor), cumin, oregano, bay leaves, and more salt if needed.
6. Add tomato sauce and 1/4 cup of water and mix well.
7. Reduce heat to low and simmer covered about 15 minutes.
8. Remove the plantains from the oven and fill them with 1/3 cup each of picadillo, then top each with 2 tbsp of cheese.
9. Return to the oven and bake until melted, about 5 minutes. Top with cilantro and serve immediately.

HAITIAN FRIED PORK WITH PLANTAINS BOWL

Griots is a rich, flavorful dish and one of Haiti's most popular, invariably served at parties and family gatherings. Cubes of pork are soaked in a sour orange marinade and then slow-roasted until tender. The tender morsels are then given a final fry in oil until delectably caramelized. This recipe uses a mixture of orange and lime juice in place of the hard-to-find sour orange juice. Also spelled grillots, griyo, griot.

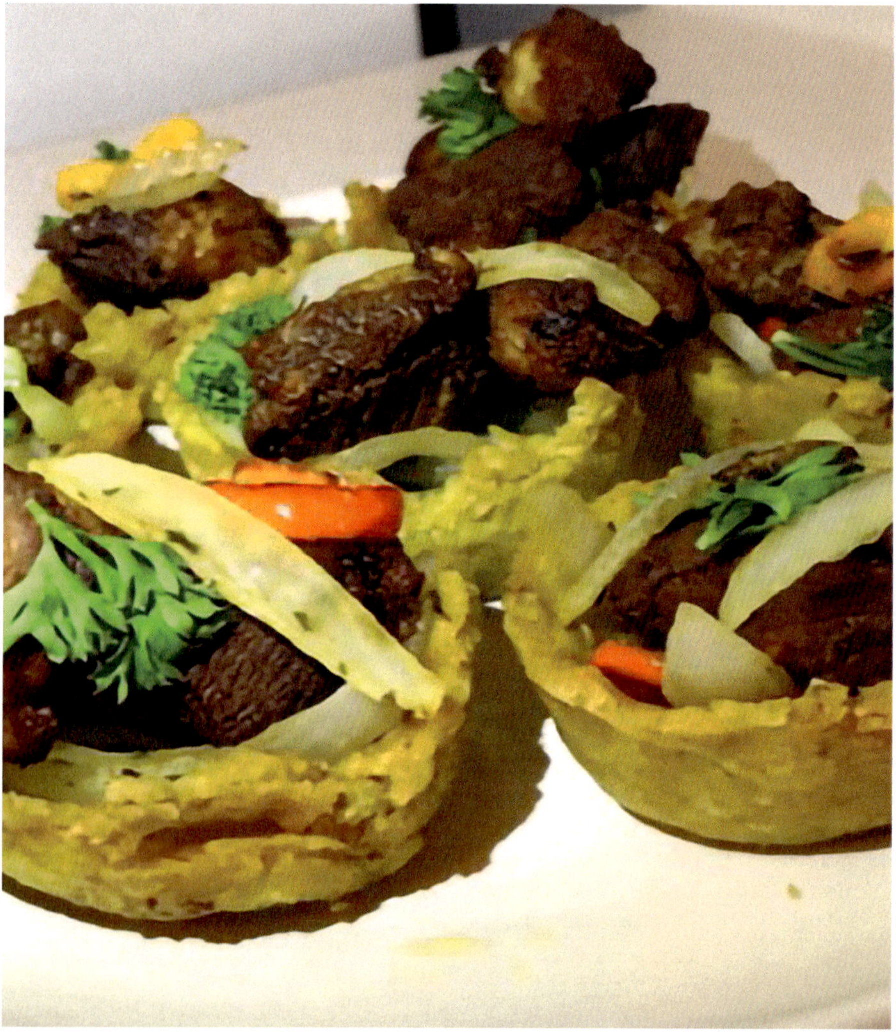

INGREDIENTS

- 4 pounds of pork shoulder, cubed
- 1 Onion, thinly sliced
- 1 green or red bell pepper, thinly sliced
- 1-2 Scotch bonnet peppers, chopped (optional)
- 2 or 3 Shallots, thinly sliced
- 3 or 4 cloves of Garlic, chopped
- 2 teaspoons of Thyme
- 2 teaspoons of salt
- 1 teaspoon of Pepper
- 2 Oranges
- 3 Limes
- ¼ cup of Oil

INSTRUCTIONS

1. Add the pork and all the other ingredients except the oil to a large, non-reactive bowl and mix together well. Refrigerate for 4 to 24 hours to let the meat soak up the marinade.
2. Oven to 375°F. Place the pork and its marinade into a large roasting pan and cover tightly with a lid or aluminum foil. Place in the oven and roast for 1 1/2 to 2 hours or until the pork is tender.
3. Remove the roasting pan from the oven. Remove any extra liquid in the pan, putting it into a saucepan, and set aside. Add the oil to the pan and stir it into the meat. Return the roasting pan to the oven and let the pork cook for 20 to 30 minutes more, stirring occasionally. Any liquid will evaporate away, and the meat will begin to fry in the oil and brown.
4. While the meat is frying in the oven, place the saucepan with the reserved liquid on the top of the stove and boil it down until it is well reduced and thickens. Remove the roasting pan from the oven and mix the reduced sauce into the browned pork. Serve hot with sos ti-malice, banan peze, and a side of pikliz.

Griots Variations

1. Use sour orange juice if you can find it. Or substitute pikliz vinegar for some of the orange and lime juice if you like.
2. Griots can also be made on the stovetop. Use a large Dutch oven with a tight-fitting lid.
3. Finely chopped scallions can be substituted for the shallots. Use four or five scallions.

HAITIAN MARINADE

Haitian marinades are a spiced batter, deep-fried fritter. Marinades are made with fish, chicken, and also vegetarian. It's quick and easy. It can also be made with cooked cod for the traditional variation of a marinade.

This goes well with banane peze (fried plantains), pikliz, and poule en sauce (stewed chicken).

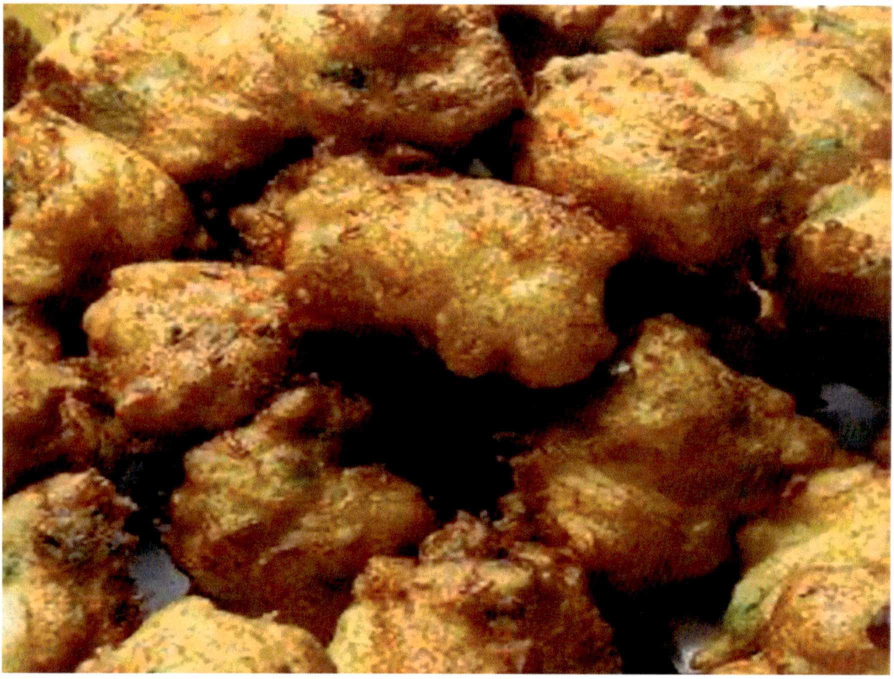

INGREDIENTS

1 egg yolk

1 cup of smoked herring or codfish

2 egg whites

1 tbsp of salt

2 scallions

2 tbsp of parsley

1 tsp each of lime juice and hot sauce

1 cup of flour

1 tbsp of baking powder

2 1/2 cups of water

1/4 cup of oil

Assemble The Following For Chicken Marinade:

3 cups flour

- 1 cup of water
- 1 tsp each of minced parsley and crushed chili pepper
- 2 tsp of baking powder
- 1 cup of cooked shredded chicken
- salt to taste
- 1 cup of vegetable oil

Prepare Vegetarian Marinade Using A Blender To Organize The Following:

- 1 minced shallot
- 1/2 chopped onion
- 1 crushed garlic clove
- 1 chopped scallion
- 2 cups of water
- 1 tsp of black pepper, parsley
- 1 tbsp of Adobo
- 2 tsp of hot sauce
- 2 eggs
- 2 tbsp of baking soda
- 1 cup of flour
- 1/2 cup of olive oil

INSTRUCTIONS

1. Combine all ingredients except oil, flour, and baking powder. Mix flour with baking powder in a separate bowl. Add flour/baking powder mixture to the rest of the ingredients to make the batter. Spoon dollops of batter into the hot oil, turning them until brown.

Assemble The Following For Chicken Marinade:

2. Stir water into flour to make the batter. Mix in chilies, parsley, and baking powder. Allow olio to stand for 60 minutes. Add chicken and salt. Spoon dollops of batter into the hot oil, turning them until brown.

Prepare Vegetarian Marinade Using A Blender To Organize The Following:

3. Blend water, shallot, onion, garlic, scallion, parsley, and Adobo. In a mixing bowl, add the rest of the ingredients plus blended ingredients to make the batter. Spoon dollops of batter into the hot oil, turning them until brown.

CHIKTAY ARANSO/ SMOKED HERRING CHIQUETAILLE

This dish needs to start being prepared at least one day in advance.

INGREDIENTS

- 1/2 cup of oil
- 1 Purple onion cut into cubes
- 2 -3 Caribbean Pepper (Scotch Bonnet Peppers)
- 1/2 cup of shallots (chopped)
- Black Pepper to taste
- NO SALT
- 4-5 smoked herrings
- 1/4 cup of white vinegar

INSTRUCTIONS

Because the smoked herring is very salted and dry (this is done to preserve the fish so that it doesn't perish), the first process will be to desalt the fish.

1. Fill a recipient of water at room temperature. Let your herring soak inside the bowl for 10 to 12 hours or simply overnight. Change the water as often as you think you should. Check for saltiness.
2. Fill a pot with water. Not too much. Just enough to cover the fish. Let it boil for 10-15 mins. You will notice that the fish will slowly open up, exposing its bone.
3. Once you're done boiling, drain the water out and start" fishing" for bones. Take out the very hard bones. Don't worry about the soft ones; they're edible. (I'm scared of fish bones, so I took out as much as I could). Tear the fish into small little pieces leaving out the skin. That part should be easy because this will tend to happen as you're taking out the bones.
4. Whisk your oil and vinegar together. Add your herring to the mixture.
5. Wash your Caribbean Peppers, throw out the seeds and cut into small pieces (do so using a glove so that you don't accidentally rub your eyes with your fingers that may have come in contact with the peppers).

6. Add peppers to the oil-vinegar-herring mixture. Add the remaining seasonings (shallots, onions, black pepper)
7. Mix well and leave in a pot over the fire for about 5 mins, stirring regularly.
8. Sometimes you may boil out too much salt (meaning that you left your herring with no salt). That actually happened while I was cooking. So, I had to add a little bit more salt.

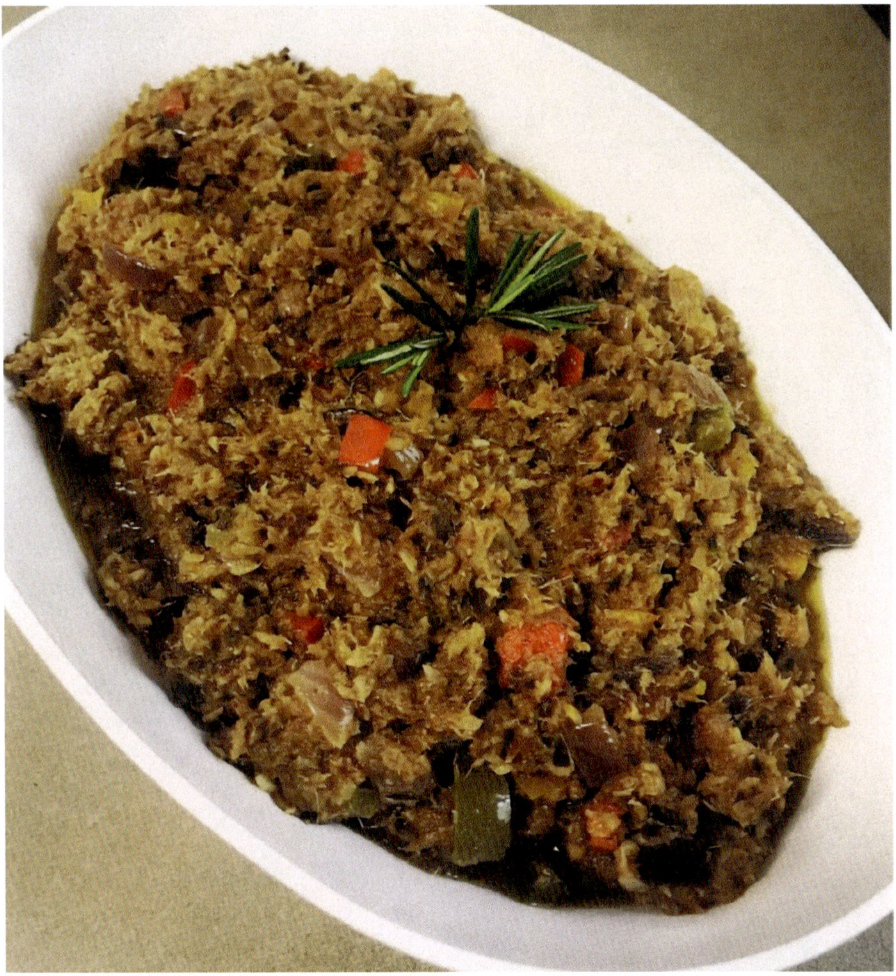

PUFF PASTRY BEEF PATTIES

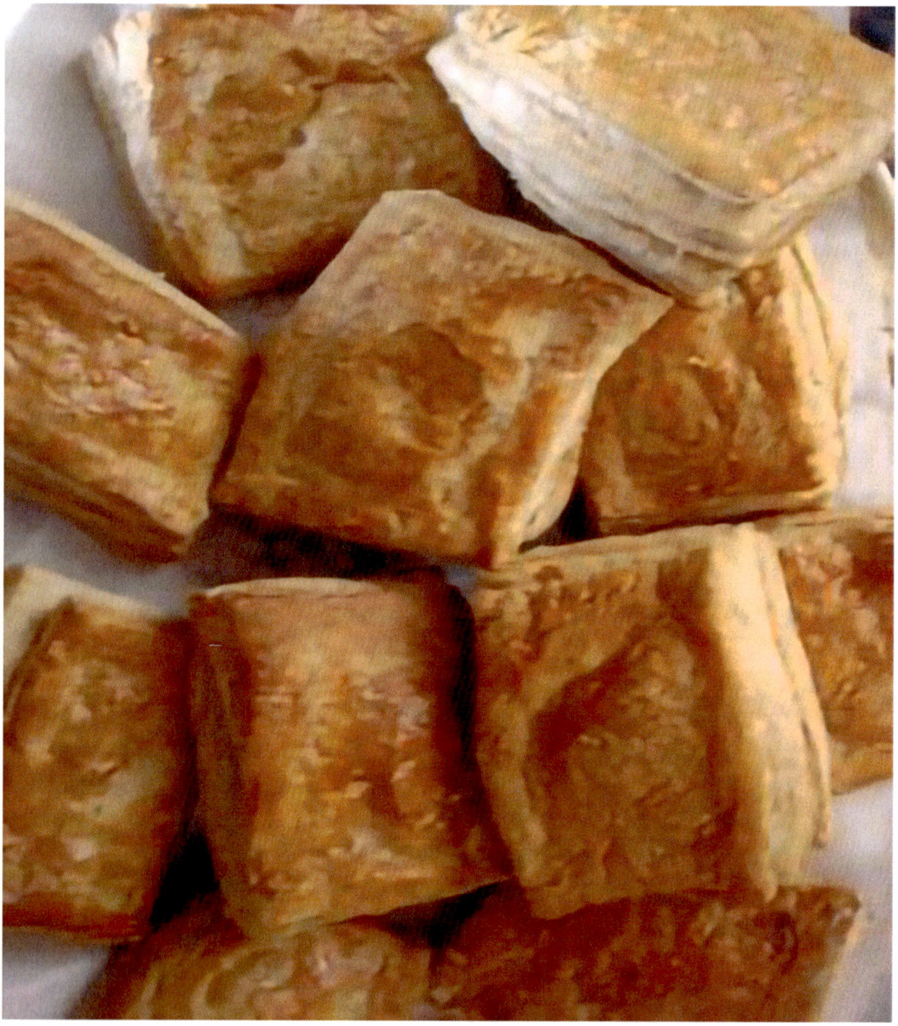

INGREDIENTS

- 1 cup of cold water
- 1 egg yolk (beaten)
- 3 cups of all-purpose flour
- 1 tsp. of salt
- Hot pepper (to taste)
- 1 tbsp. of vinegar (white)
- 1/4 cup of butter (softened)
- 1 cup of vegetable shortening
- 1 lb of cooked ground beef (or another kind of meat you favor)
- 2 tsp. of parsley
- 1 clove of garlic (chopped)
- 2 shallots (chopped)
- 1 tbsp. of broth

INSTRUCTIONS

1. Make a paste with the hot pepper, garlic, parsley, and shallots.
2. Season cooked meat with seasoning paste and broth.
3. Cook for ten minutes over medium heat in a covered pot while stirring constantly.
4. When all the liquid has been cooked off, the filling will be ready.
5. In a large mixing bowl, add flour and make a hole in its center. Into the hole, pour water and add the salt. Using a spoon to mix, combine ingredients without kneading.
6. Refrigerate dough for 30 minutes.
7. Mix shortening and butter in a bowl.
8. Roll dough into 1/4 inch thick rectangle then spread with half of the shortening mix.
9. Fold an edge over the middle and spread the remaining shortening on this section. Then fold over the last section and roll the dough to a thickness of 1/4 inch. Fold into thirds and roll again repeat, then refrigerate overnight.
10. Roll dough to a thickness of 1/2 an inch and then cut into rounds of 1 1/2 inches.
11. Place a spoonful of meat mixture on one side and fold over the other side, pressing the ends together.
12. Place on a baking sheet, brush with egg yolks, and bake in the oven with a pan of water on the rack below at 4000 F for 30 minutes. Turn the oven down to 3000 F and bake for another 20 minutes or until patties are golden brown.

02
SALADE

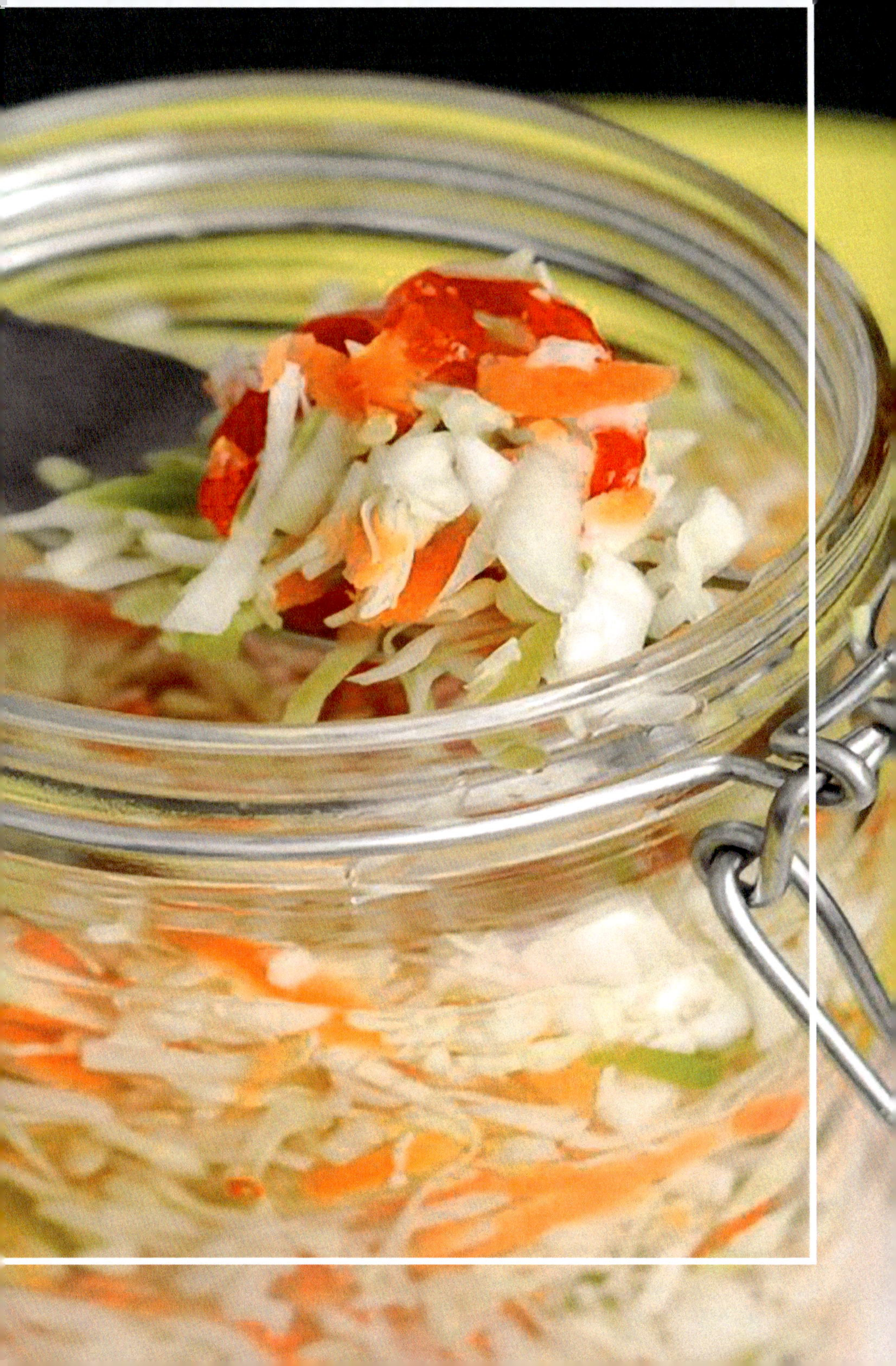

HAITIAN SALAD RUSE

INGREDIENTS

4 potatoes

1 – 2 carrots

1 large beet

1/2 cup of sweet peas

¼ cup of onion minced

1/3 cup of green bell pepper diced

1/3 teaspoon of garlic powder

2 – 3 tablespoons of mayonnaise

Salt and pepper to taste

INSTRUCTIONS

1. Peel potatoes and add to a large saucepan with water and boil until fully cooked but not too soft.
2. Remove from water, cut in cubes, and set aside. While the potatoes are cooking, peel and cut the carrots in small cubes and set aside to cool. In another saucepan, add carrots and peas with a little bit of water. Bring to a boil and cook thoroughly.
3. Remove from water and set aside to cool. In another saucepan, add beet and cook thoroughly.
4. When cooked, peel and cut in cubes and set aside to cool. In a large bowl, add potatoes, beet, carrots, peas, onion, green bell pepper, mayonnaise, garlic powder, salt, and pepper to taste. Stir to mix and serve immediately.

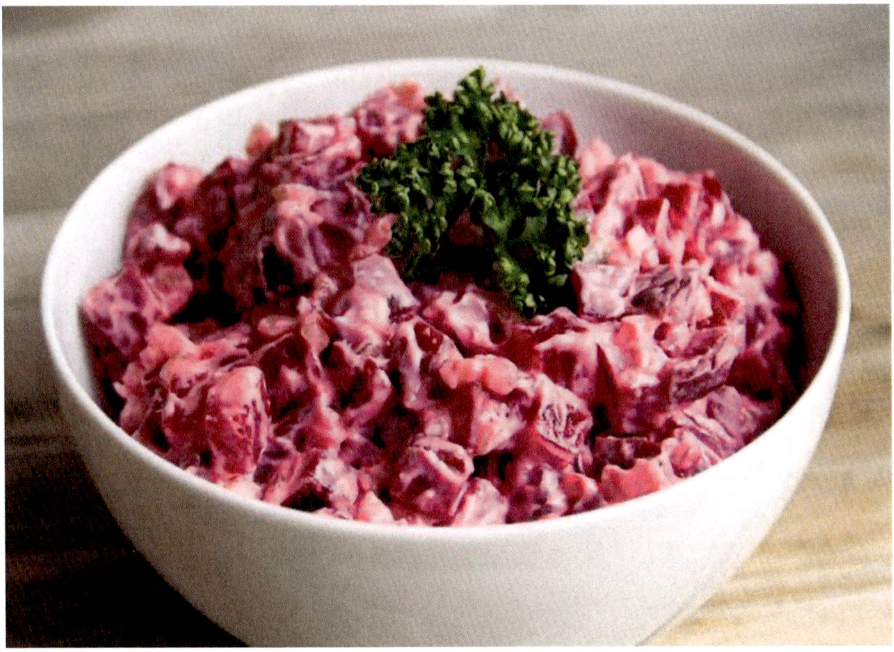

CARROT AND APPLE SLAW

INGREDIENTS

10 oz. Grimmway Farms Shredded Carrots

4 cups of Granny Smith apples cut into matchstick-sized slices

1 cup of raisins

1/4 cup of mayonnaise

3 tbsp of nonfat Greek Yogurt

3 tbsp of rice vinegar

3 tbsp of honey

1/2 tsp of salt

1/2 tsp of celery seeds

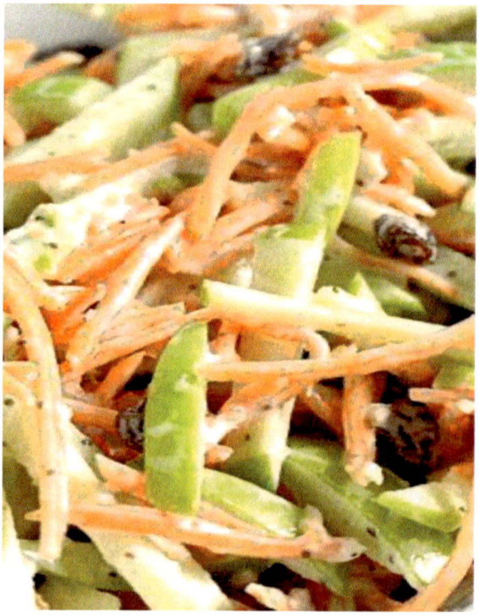

INSTRUCTIONS

1. In a medium-sized bowl, whisk mayonnaise, Greek yogurt, rice vinegar, honey, salt, and celery seeds
2. Add carrots, apple, and raisins
3. Toss in the dressing
4. Enjoy!

CARIBBEAN POTATO SALAD

INGREDIENTS

2 pounds of Yukon gold potatoes, skin left on and whole

2 eggs

2 tablespoons of red vinegar

1/4 cup of olive oil

1/4 cup of black olives, pitted and diced

1/2 cup of red onion, diced

3 tablespoons of Italian parsley, finely minced

kosher salt, to taste

fresh cracked black pepper, to taste

INSTRUCTIONS

1. Place the potatoes and eggs into a large pan with cold water. Sprinkle with a little salt.
2. Bring to boil over high heat, then lower to simmer. Cook until the potatoes are fork-tender; it took about 20 minutes with the size of potatoes I had.
3. Drain into a colander.
4. Rinse both the eggs and potatoes under very cold water. Then let sit in the colander for an hour – this step eliminates unnecessary water.
5. Cut the potatoes into bite-size pieces and place into a bowl.
6. Sprinkle the red vinegar over the top of the potatoes and let sit for 15 minutes.
7. Dice the eggs.
8. Gently fold in the olives, diced eggs, red onion, and parsley. Drizzle over the olive oil and fold again.
9. Season to taste with salt and pepper.
10. Cover and then place into the refrigerator for at least 4 hours or overnight.

HAITIAN SPICY COLESLAW

The Caribbean is flooded with pepper sauces and condiments of all kinds, as it's simply part of our culinary culture. The textures, heat level, ingredients, ways of preserving, and overall vibrancy of them all are unique to the maker and individual island. In Trinidad and Tobago, you'll find a lot of chutneys and amchars, while in Barbados, you'll hear the locals boast about their pepper sauce. As someone who considers myself an aficionado of anything hot and spicy, it must be said that Haitian Pikliz is at the top of my list when it comes to spicy condiments.

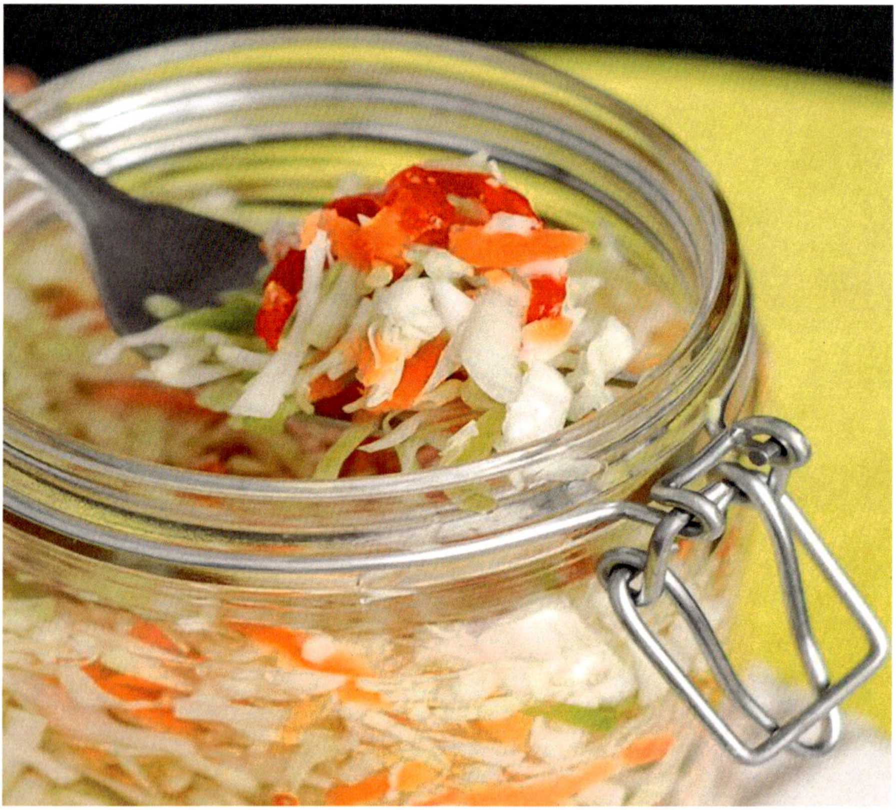

The slight crunch of the vegetables, the heat from the thinly sliced scotch bonnet peppers, and the flavors the vinegar (takes on), which is used to bring it all together, is just outstanding (after marinating for about a week or so). This recipe is dedicated to the beautiful people of Haiti.

INGREDIENTS

- 2 cups of shredded cabbage
- 1 large carrot
- 1 cup of bell pepper (green, orange, red)
- 1 onion
- 2 scallions
- 6 scotch bonnet peppers
- 4 cloves of garlic
- 1 teaspoon of salt
- 12-14 peppercorns
- 2 cups of vinegar (see note)
- 1/2 lime juice
- * 4 cloves (traditionally used)

INSTRUCTIONS

1. This is a very simple recipe to put together as it involves a couple of steps and some patience (to marinate). Start off by slicing the cabbage very thinly, the same for all the other ingredients. You may be tempted to use a food processor, but I would suggest you don't. The food processor may overwork the vegetables, and you won't get that unique size/shape pikliz is supposed to have. Grate the carrot and dice the garlic very fine.
2. Place all the sliced ingredients in a large bowl large enough so you can easily mix everything easily without spilling all over the place. Also mix in the salt, peppercorns, and cloves.
3. Get a fairly large glass bottle and pack in everything, then all you have to do is top with the vinegar, cover, and set aside to marinate. You can certainly begin using right away, but if you give it about five days to marinate and really take on the flavors of everything, you'll be rewarded with the best pikliz you've ever had.
4. Since we used vinegar as the base, it will act as a preservative, so you don't have to worry about it going wrong if you don't store it in the fridge. However, if you do store it in the fridge, it can last months. But be aware that some of the heat will be lost the longer it stays in the fridge. Now, if only I had some Griot to accompany this Pikliz!

Note:

Add enough vinegar to cover the ingredients in the storage container. Allow it to marinate for about 5 days before use. I was out of cloves, but it's a traditional ingredient used in making this lovely pickle, so I would recommend using it.

03
SOUPS

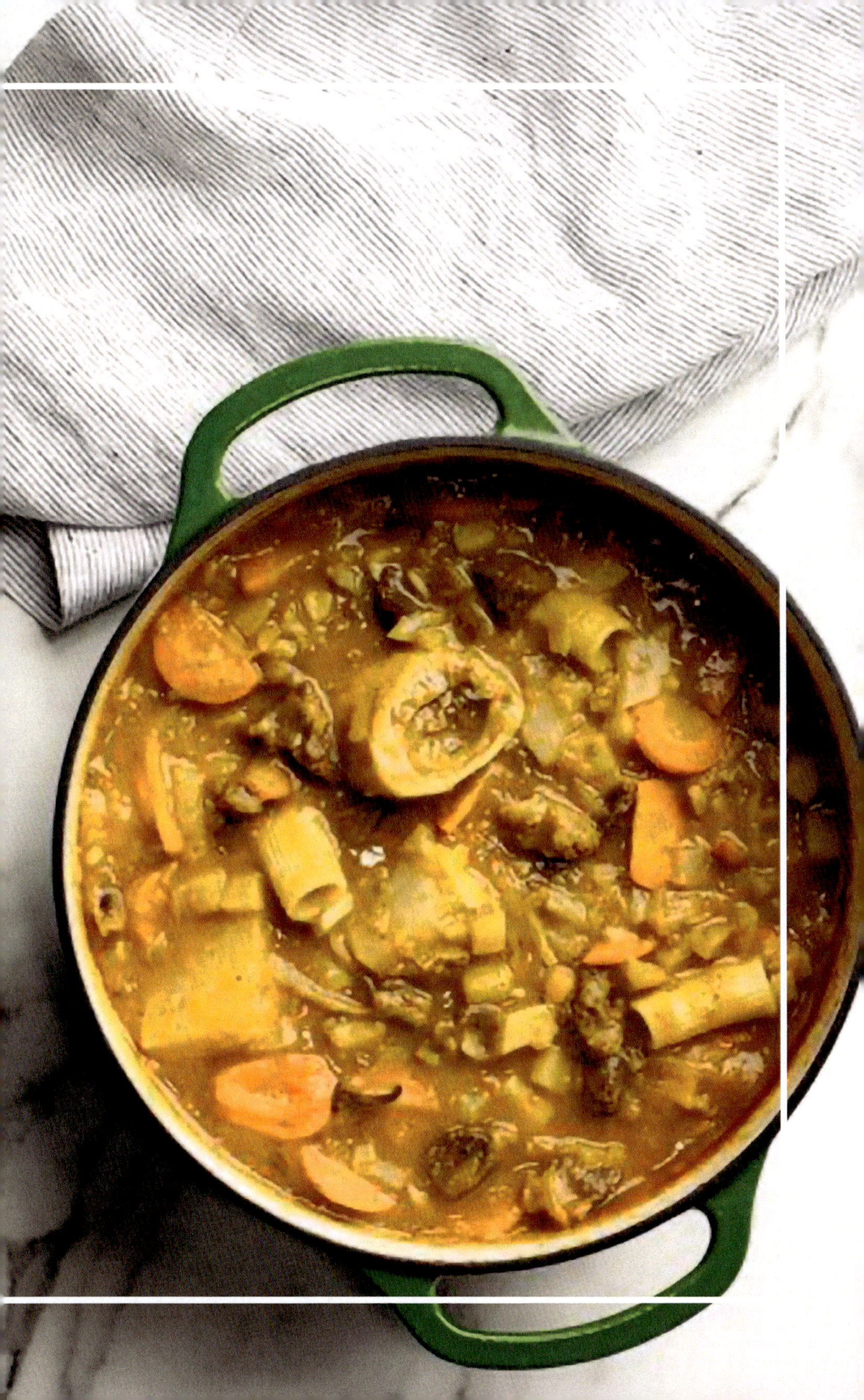

HAITIAN PUMPKIN SOUP

Soup Joumou is served every year on the 1st of January as the Haitian nation celebrates its Independence. It is one of the most savored foods, as it is a rarity. Deliciously prepared to one's taste, but the base is squash. Extremely filling, but yet, the enjoyment of the sensational flavors with the proudness of freedom makes this dish a unique experience that one must share.

The number one and main reason that makes this soup so special to Haitians, is that it is a reminder of their struggles and victory. During slavery, Haitian slaves were not allowed to enjoy this soup as it was only to be prepared for the slave masters. Therefore, on January 1, 1804, Haiti's Independence Day, the newly freed Haitians celebrated their freedom with SOUP JOUMOU.

No matter where you are in the world, if you are Haitian or Haitian descendant, you are most likely celebrating the New Year with a bowl of Soup Joumou. It is said you cannot make soup joumou without love, patience, and a smile on your face.

Haitian Soup Joumou is rich and hearty. It is not as thick as the traditional squash soup you will find in most places. It is filled with vegetables, as we call it Viv. It is hearty and meaty. It is the type of soup that literally fills you up all day. It is starchy but yet healthy. It is savory and sometimes made with a hint of sweetness, depending on the individual who is making it.

It is our beloved and most delicious soup for many reasons. For example, to make soup joumou, the meat is marinated overnight (or two). Traditionally, a combination of the following meat is included: beef, chicken, goat meat, and pork meat.

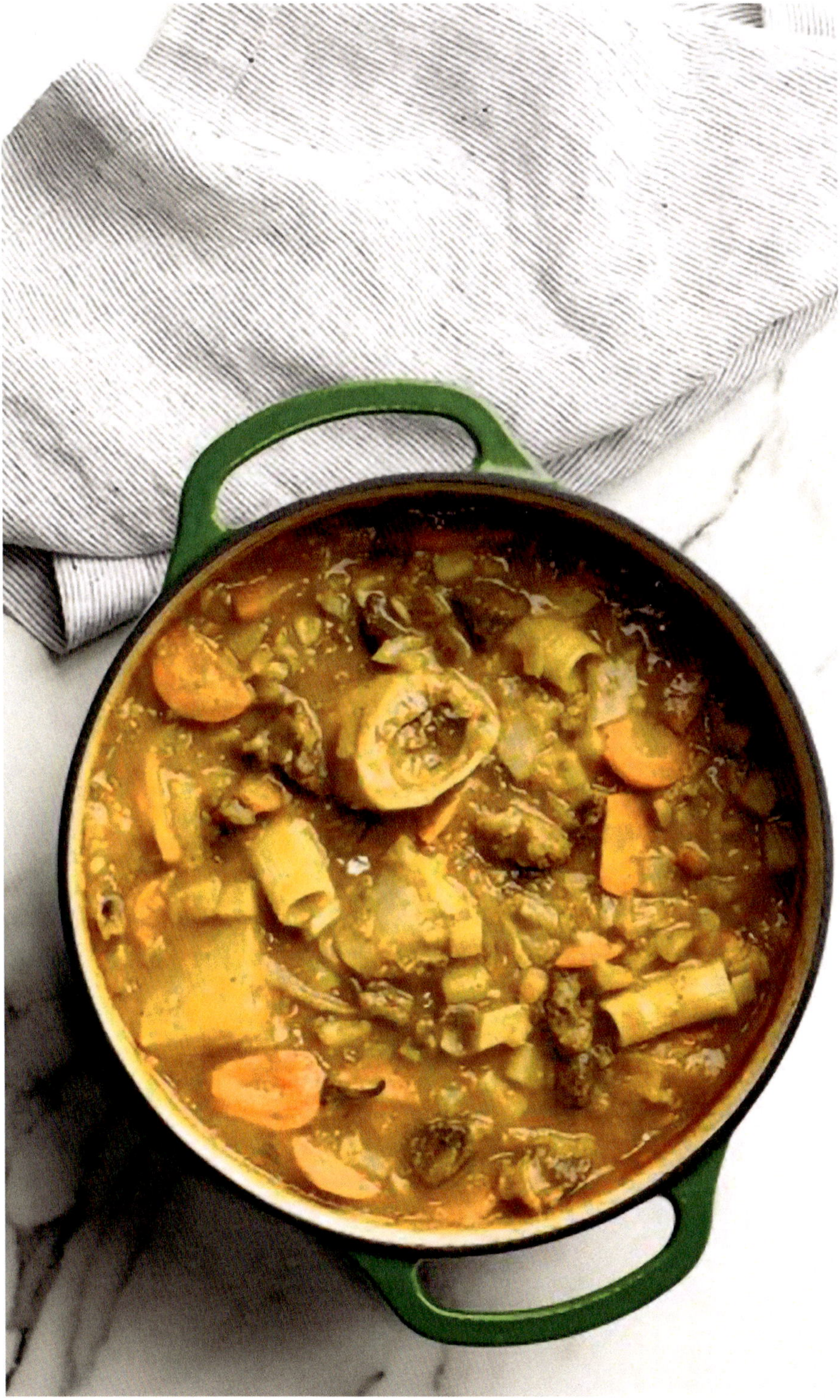

INGREDIENTS

1 cup, plus 1 tablespoon of distilled white vinegar, divided

1 pound of beef shank, meat cut off bones into 1″ cubes

1 pound of stew beef (preferably chuck) cut into 1″ cubes

1 cup of Epis Seasoning Base

3 tablespoons of fresh lime juice (from about 1 lime)

1 tablespoon of seasoned salt

15 cups of beef or vegetable broth, divided

1 pound of beef bones

1 medium of calabaza squash (about 2 pounds), peeled, cubed, or 2 pounds defrosted frozen cubed calabaza squash, or 1 butternut squash (about 2 pounds), peeled, cut into 2″ chunks

3 large russet potatoes (about 2 pounds), finely chopped

3 carrots (about 1 pound), sliced

1/2 small green cabbage (about 1 pound), very thinly sliced

1 medium onion, sliced

1 celery stalk, coarsely chopped

1 leek, white and pale-green parts only, finely chopped

2 small turnips, finely chopped

1 green Scotch bonnet or habanero chile

1 1/2 cups of rigatoni

6 whole cloves

1 teaspoon of garlic powder

1 teaspoon of onion powder

2 1/2 teaspoons of kosher salt, plus more

1/2 teaspoon of freshly ground black pepper, plus more

Pinch of cayenne pepper, plus more

1 parsley sprig (optional)

1 thyme sprig (optional)

2 tablespoons of olive oil

1 tablespoon of unsalted butter

Crusty bread (for serving)

A very large stockpot

INSTRUCTIONS

1. Pour 1 cup of vinegar into a large bowl. Swish beef shank and stew beef in vinegar to rinse. Transfer beef to a colander and rinse with water.
2. Stir Epis Seasoning Base, lime juice, and seasoned salt in another large bowl. Add beef, toss to coat, and let marinate at least 30 minutes, preferably overnight.
3. Heat 5 cups of broth in a very large stockpot over medium. Add marinated beef and bones, cover, and simmer until meat is beginning to soften about 40 minutes.
4. Add squash to pot on top of beef, cover, and return to a simmer. Cook until squash is fork-tender, 20–25 minutes. Using tongs or a slotted spoon, transfer squash to a blender. Add 4 cups of broth and purée until smooth. Return to the pot and bring to a simmer.
5. Add potatoes, carrots, cabbage, onion, celery, leek, turnips, chile, rigatoni, cloves, garlic powder, onion powder, 2 1/2 tsp. of salt, 1/2 tsp. of pepper, a pinch of cayenne, parsley, if using, thyme, if using, and remaining 6 cups of broth. Simmer uncovered, until pasta and vegetables are tender, 30–35 minutes.
6. Add oil, butter, and remaining 1 Tbsp. of Vinegar. Reduce heat to medium-low and simmer until beef is very tender, 15–20 minutes more.
7. Taste and adjust seasonings. Divide soup among bowls and serve with bread alongside.

BRAISED OXTAIL RAGU

If you've never had oxtail before, I highly recommend it. This is something that you should be having, at least on occasion. It's not one of those foods that you need to have on a regular basis. However, it should be something that you have when you want to treat yourself to something a little different.

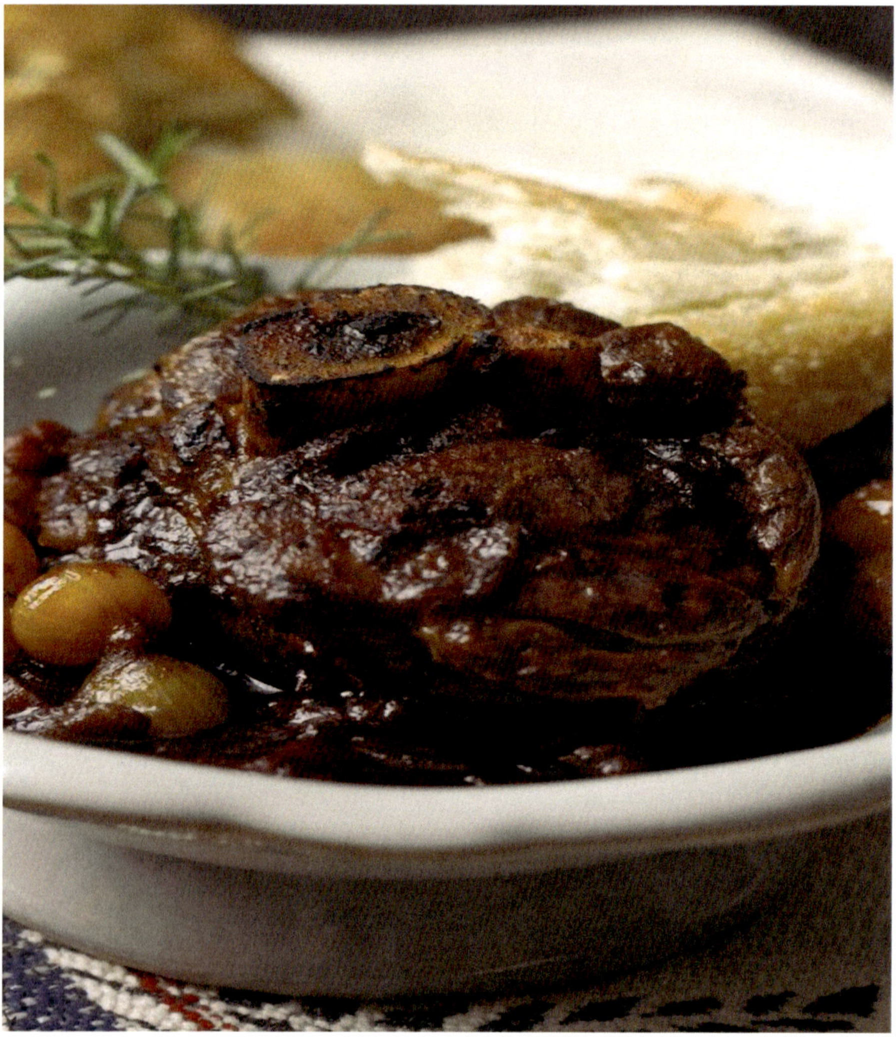

INGREDIENTS

4 to 5 pounds of oxtail, cut into 3-inch pieces at the butcher

Salt and freshly ground black pepper

Flour, for dredging

1/4 cup of olive oil

1 medium yellow onion, chopped

1 large carrot, chopped

3 whole celery ribs, chopped

1 (28-ounces) can plum tomatoes, crushed

3 cups of dry red wine

2 rosemary sprigs

2 thyme sprigs

2 bay leaves

4 cloves of garlic, peeled and smashed

1/4 teaspoon of freshly grated nutmeg

INSTRUCTIONS

1. Preheat the oven to 300°F.
2. Pat the meat dry with paper towels then dust with the flour, tapping off any excess. Season with salt and pepper on all sides.
3. Place a 6-quart Dutch oven or other heavy-bottomed, oven-safe pot with a tight-fitting lid over medium-high heat. Add the oil, and when glistening, add the meat (metal tongs come in handy here) and sear on all sides, about 8 to 10 minutes. Work in batches if necessary to avoid overcrowding.
4. Transfer the meat to a plate. Add onion, carrot, and celery and cook, frequently stirring, until browned, about 5 to 7 minutes. Add the tomatoes with their juices, wine, rosemary, thyme, bay leaves, garlic, and nutmeg. Bring to a boil for 5 minutes.
5. Add the meat and enough water to just barely cover the meat. Return to a boil, then cover the pot and transfer it to the oven. Cook for 3 to 4 hours, until the meat is fork-tender and falling off the bones.
6. Remove the pot from the oven and transfer the pieces of meat to a plate. Skim any visible fat from the surface of the sauce. Pick the meat from the bones, pulling away and discarding any pieces of fat, and then return the meat to the pan. Pluck out the bay leaves, and sprigs of rosemary and thyme. Season the sauce with salt and pepper.
7. Serve atop gnocchi or any pasta meant to withstand a hearty sauce. The ragù can be made a few days ahead; keep covered and refrigerated, then reheat over medium-low heat.

RECIPE NOTES

This is a hearty, chunky sauce. If you prefer something more uniform in texture, blend a portion or all of the sauce in a blender.

JAMAICAN STEW PEAS

This hearty Red Peas Soup recipe is so flavorful, comforting, and warming. It is perfect for chilly evenings. Red beans cooked in a flavorful herb-infused coconut broth with potato, carrots, yam, and dumplings.

INGREDIENTS

1 lb. pigs' tail or stew beef, seasoned

2 cups of dry red kidney beans

1 medium onion, chopped

3 stalks of scallion (green onions), chopped

2 sprigs of thyme, chopped

1 green bell pepper, chopped

3 cloves of garlic, chopped

10 pimento seeds, crushed or 1 tsp of allspice

8 cups of water

1 can of coconut milk

1 scotch bonnet pepper or 1/4 tsp of red pepper flakes

Spinners

Ingredients for Spinners (Dumplings)

cup of flour

1/4 tsp of salt

Just about 1/3 cup of water

INSTRUCTIONS

Make Spinners

1. In a small bowl, add the flour and salt and whisk it. Add the water a little at a time and knead to form a smooth dough. Cover and Set aside for later to add to the Jamaican Stew Peas Recipe.

Make Jamaican Stew Peas

2. Rinse the beans with some water and drain. Put the beans in a large pot/skillet with the garlic, pimento berries or allspice, pig's tail, and 6 cups of water. Let it cook until both beans and meat are tender, just about 1 hour and 20 minutes. Add the onion, 2 stalks of scallion, thyme, bell pepper, 2 cups of water, can of milk and bring it to a boil.

3. Break apart the dough into small pieces and roll between your palms to make spinner (dumplings), and add to the pot. Add the scotch bonnet pepper or red pepper flakes and black pepper. Continue to stir the mixture, so the spinners won't stick to the bottom of the pot as it cooks.
4. Allow to simmer on medium-low for about 40 minutes or until it thickens to your desire. Stir to make sure nothing is sticking at the bottom but be careful not to burst the pepper.
5. After about 30 minutes of cooking on medium-low, add the remaining 1 stalk of scallion (chopped) and stir. Turn the heat on semi-low.
6. Taste and see if it's to your desire. If it is not to your desire, add some salt. Remove the scotch bonnet pepper and thyme from the pot before serving. Best served with some white rice. Enjoy.

Notes:

1. *Not everyone uses coconut milk in their Jamaican Stew Peas Recipe. I used it because of the flavor it gives, and it helps to thicken the sauce. Others mix a small amount of flour with water and add to the liquid to thicken the sauce.*
2. *Please remove the scotch bonnet pepper and thyme before serving.*

HAITIAN TCHAKA SOUP RECIPE

Tchaka is a Haitian delicacy made from different grain ingredients. The dish is a combination of red beans together with dried corn, salt-cured pig foot, and traditional spices. The delicacy is one of the most treasured recipes that have continued to define the culture of Haitian Creole.

Tchaka Soup is a dish that has continued to attract the attention of many people who visit Haiti. Today, we'll take you through the Tchaka soup preparation process. First, let's get to know more about Haitians' dining culture.

The people of Haiti have adopted the typical French dining culture. This is as a result of French colonization. Yet, there are many indigenous dishes and dining practices that have survived for ages. Many of Haiti's dining cultures have melted together in a pot of history. For instance, some dining cultures starting with the indigenous people living in the region at the time, have mixed with that of slaves who were held there to support Haiti's plantation economy. However, this melted pot serves to further enrich the Haitian's culture and traditions, and their Tasty Tchaka Soup is a proof.

Their cuisine is a starch-filled diet that is occasionally accompanied by meat (pork and mutton). Almost all the dishes of Haitian origin have pepper in them. Apart from pork and goat-meat, Haitian main dishes have seafood. It's no surprise, Haiti is located in the Caribbean, where lobsters are readily available and are valued to be the source of proteins for the natives.

INGREDIENTS

- 12 ounces bag of dried cut corn
- 12 ounces bag of dried red beans
- 12 ounces bag of dried chickpeas
- 2 pounds of smoked turkey neck or smoked pork
- 1 yellow onion, rough chopped
- 4 cloves of garlic
- 1 stalk of celery
- 2 (14.5 ounces) cans of coconut milk
- 2 packs of frozen cooked squash
- salt and pepper to taste
- garlic powder
- onion powder
- 2 packs of sazon seasoning
- 1 big bunch of parsley

INSTRUCTIONS

1. Boil beans, corn, and chickpeas in unsalted water, in three separate stock pots (because each requires a different amount of time to fully cook), for about 2 hours until tender. Add additional water to the stockpot as necessary to prevent the corn and beans from burning.
2. 2. If you're using pork, clean all of the excess fat off of the Braise the meat in a pressure cooker for 30 minutes, or until the meat is tender.
3. Rough chop the onion, garlic, and celery. Transfer to a blender and pulse until pureed. Set aside.
4. When the corn, beans, and chickpeas are fully cooked, combine all (including the cooking liquid) in one large 12-quart stockpot.
5. When the meat is tender, remove from its liquid and transfer into the stockpot. Pour the liquid into a fat separator. If you don't own one, then pour the liquid into a container, passing through a strainer and catching all of the excess skin and fat. Pour this strained liquid into the stockpot.
6. Add the coconut milk and frozen squash to the pot. The squash quickly will defrost during cooking. After the squash melts, add additional water until the soup reaches almost to the rim of the pot. The contents of the pot should not overflow when the lid is placed on the pot.
7. 7. Carefully stir in the vegetable puree, all of the seasoning, and a tied bunch of parsley to the stockpot.
8. Let everything simmer on medium heat until all of the spices have penetrated into the soup, about 30 minutes. You can turn the heat down to low and simmer for an additional 1 hour and REALLY let the flavor of the soup develop.
9. Serve hot with French butter bread. ENJOY!

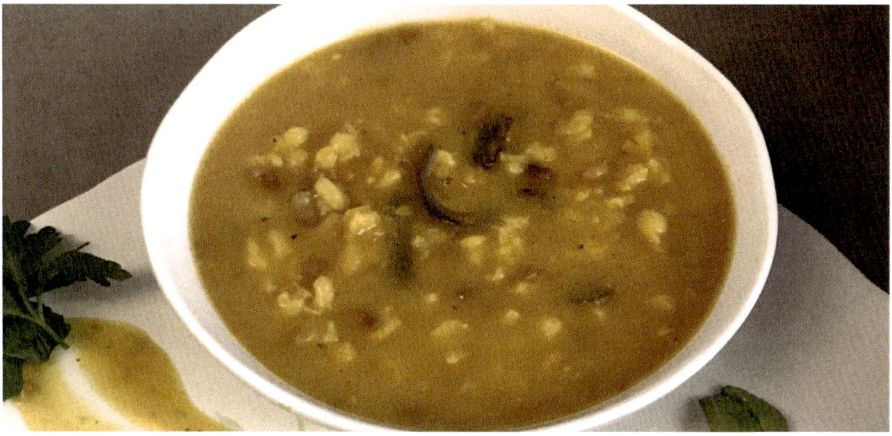

JAMAICAN CURRY GOAT

Jamaican Curry Goat is an insanely delicious, slow-cooked Jamaican Spiced Curry that is full of flavor and tender to the bone! An absolutely must-make Jamaican food! So easy to make with minimal prep.

INGREDIENTS

- 3- 3 1/2 pounds of goat meat (cut in chunks)
- ¼- ½ cup of cooking oil
- 2 teaspoons of minced garlic
- 1 medium onion sliced
- 4-5 tablespoons of curry powder
- 1- 2 teaspoons of white pepper
- 1-2 teaspoons of fresh thyme
- 2 green onions sliced
- 2-3 medium potatoes
- 1 carrot
- 1 tablespoon of tomato paste
- 1 scotch bonnet pepper (adjust to suit taste buds or replace with any hot pepper)
- 1 tablespoon of Bouillon powder (optional)
- Salt to taste

INSTRUCTIONS

1. Clean the meat with lime and lemon juice, boil some hot water with lime juice and parsley. Add the clean meat into the hot boiling water and drain the water, I usually add some of my good Haitian seasonings the night before, or you can also let it rest up to two hours before cooking it.
2. In a large pot, heat oil over medium heat until hot, and then add the goat meat sauté, stirring, frequently, any browned bits off the bottom of the pot, until the goat is brown.
3. Then add curry, stir for about 1-2 minutes. Add the carrots so it can cook with the meat.
4. Add the garlic, white pepper, onions, thyme, tomato paste, adobo, paprika, and black pepper, scallions (green onions), and scotch bonnet pepper stir for about a minute.
5. Then pour in just enough water to cover the goat and bring to a boil and let it simmer until tender (depending on the goat size and preference) about 2 hours or more, stirring the saucepan occasionally and adding more water as needed.
6. About 15-20 minutes before you remove from the stove, add potatoes and bouillon powder. Continue cooking until potatoes are tender; if you want a really thick curry goat, let the potatoes cook even more.
7. You may adjust the thickness of soup with water or stock.

CURRY CHICKEN RECIPE

This authentic Caribbean family curry chicken recipe has a list of spicy and tasty ingredients that, when combined, will give you the best curry chicken recipe you will ever taste.

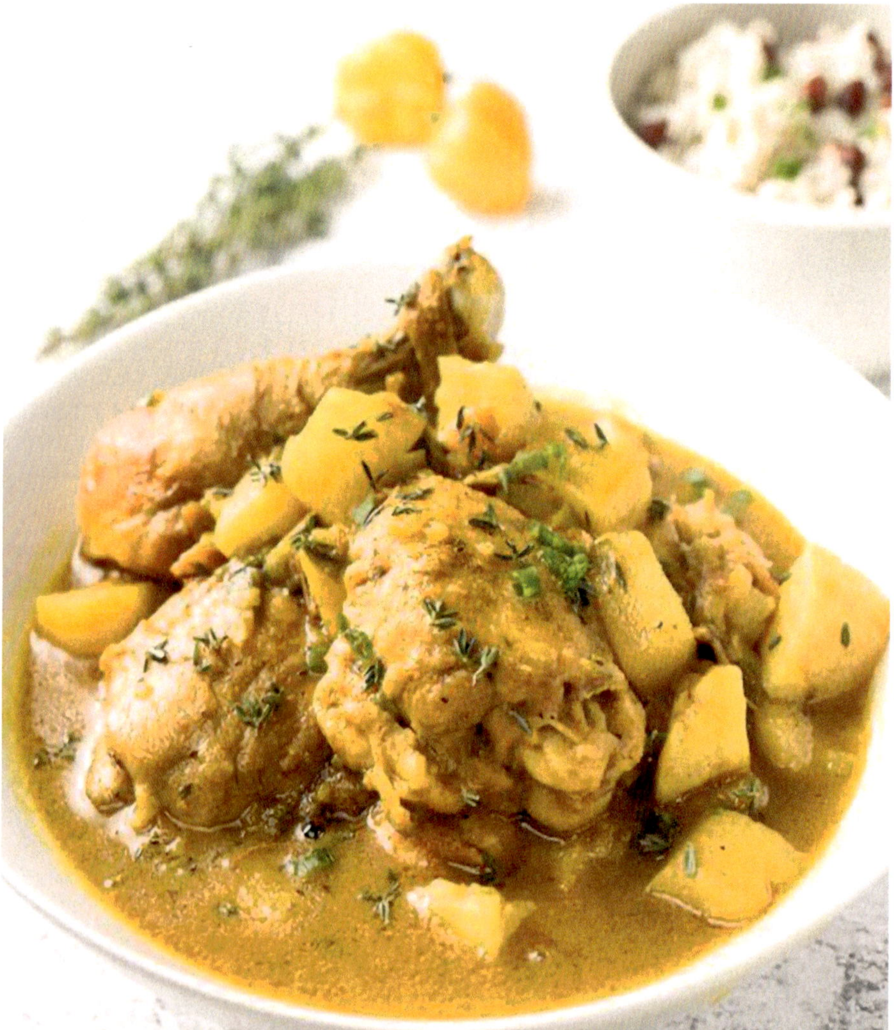

INGREDIENTS

- 3 1/2 pounds of chicken
- 1/4 cups of Vinegar
- 3 stalks of green onion, chopped
- 1 medium onion, chopped
- 4 cloves of garlic, chopped
- 1 tsp of black pepper
- 1 cup of chopped potato
- 1/4 of diced carrots
- 1/4 cup of diced Green Bell Pepper
- 2 tsp of Seasons Ghosted Curry Spice Blend
- 3 tsp of Oil
- 1 tsp of ginger, grated
- 3 1/2 cups of water

INSTRUCTIONS

1. Cut chicken into bite-size pieces and wash in a mixture of White Vinegar and water.
2. Season chicken with chopped green onion, onion, garlic, black pepper, Seasons Ghosted Curry Spice Blend. Cover and allow to marinate in the refrigerator for about 1 hour or overnight.
3. Heat oil in a heavy skillet, add 2 tsp of Seasons Ghosted Curry Spice Blend and the grated ginger, garlic, and allow to "burn" for about 45 seconds on medium heat.
4. Add the seasoned chicken, chopped potatoes, diced carrots and cook stirring for about 5-10 minutes
5. Add diced bell peppers when the chicken is close to cooked.

Notes:

1. *After five minutes, remove the lid and check if the chicken and potatoes are cooked. If not, you might want to add a bit of water to the chicken if needed. No more than 1/4 of a cup.*
2. *Add bell peppers when the chicken is close to cooked.*
3. *Add salt to taste*

JAMAICAN BROWN STEW CHICKEN

Brown Stew Chicken is a classic Jamaican stew made with chicken, vegetables, and a heavy amount of aromatic spices. The end result is a tender chicken, flavorful and rich brown stew gravy, and a wonderfully scented kitchen

INGREDIENTS

Marinade

- 3 lbs. chicken thighs washed and cleaned as instructed in the post
- 2 tsp of Himalayan pink salt
- 1 tsp of black pepper
- 3 medium-sized scallions sliced
- 2 tsp of coconut palm sugar
- 4 cloves of garlic minced
- 1/4-1/2 tsp of browning sauce

Yard Style Gravy

- 2 tbsp of coconut oil
- 1 medium-sized onion sliced
- 1 small red bell pepper
- 1 small green bell pepper
- A thumb-sized piece ginger
- 2 pimento berries or 1/4 tsp of allspice
- 1/2 tbsp of dried thyme or 3 sprigs of fresh thyme
- 1 tbsp of organic tomato puree
- 1 tsp of hot pepper sauce
- 2 cups of hot water

INSTRUCTIONS

1. Place the chicken thighs with all of the ingredients for the marinade into a large bowl and rub the entire marinade into the chicken, then store in the refrigerator overnight.
2. Preheat the oven at 230 degrees Celsius (450 degrees F) or gas mark 8.
3. Scrap off the excess marinade and store in the refrigerator. Proceed to put the chicken in the oven in a roasting pan and roast for 20-25 minutes until brown, making sure to turn over halfway through.
4. Once browned, remove from the oven and set aside.

5. Heat a large frying pan with the coconut oil on medium heat and add the onions, sautéing for 1-2 minutes until translucent.
6. Then add the bell peppers, ginger, pimento (allspice), dried thyme, tomato puree, and hot pepper sauce.
7. Flip the pan - stir and fold the entire contents.
8. Now add the chicken with a tablespoon of or two of the drippings and scrap the rest of the marinade, which was stored in the refrigerator into the pan.
9. Finally, pour in the two cups of water and stir.
10. Reduce the heat to low, cover pan with the lid, and allow to slowly simmer for 30 minutes.
11. The water levels will reduce by half and thicken slightly into a rich brown sauce as it simmers. Check the pan to see if any oil is suspended on the surface. If so, skim this off with a spoon.
12. Once the gravy has formed, remove from heat and serve accordingly.

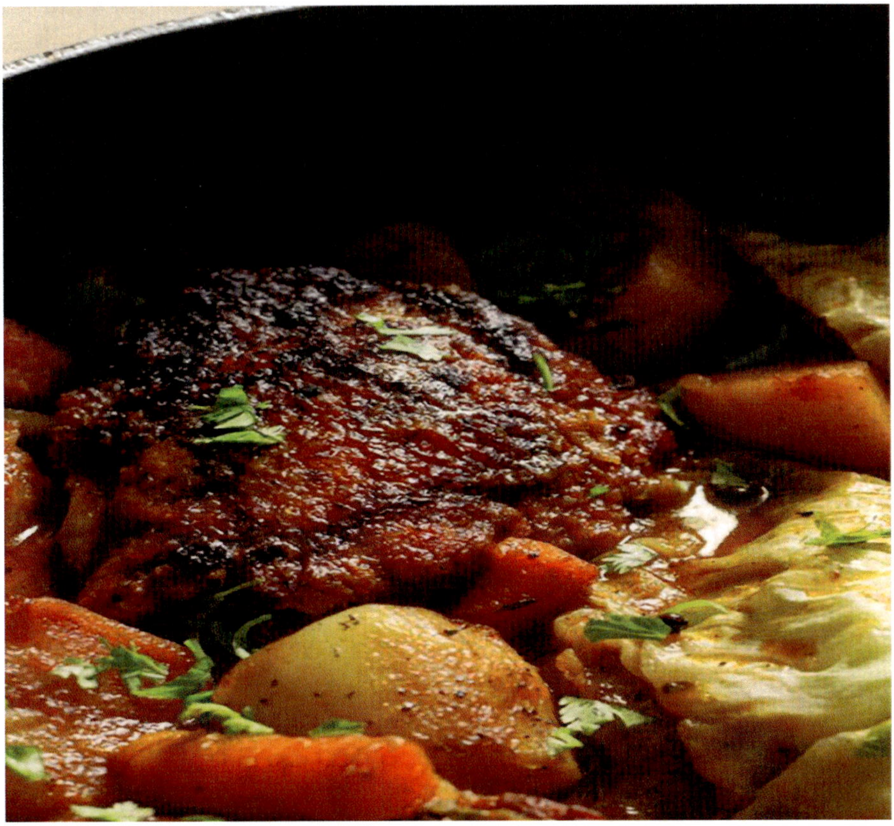

04
ENTREE

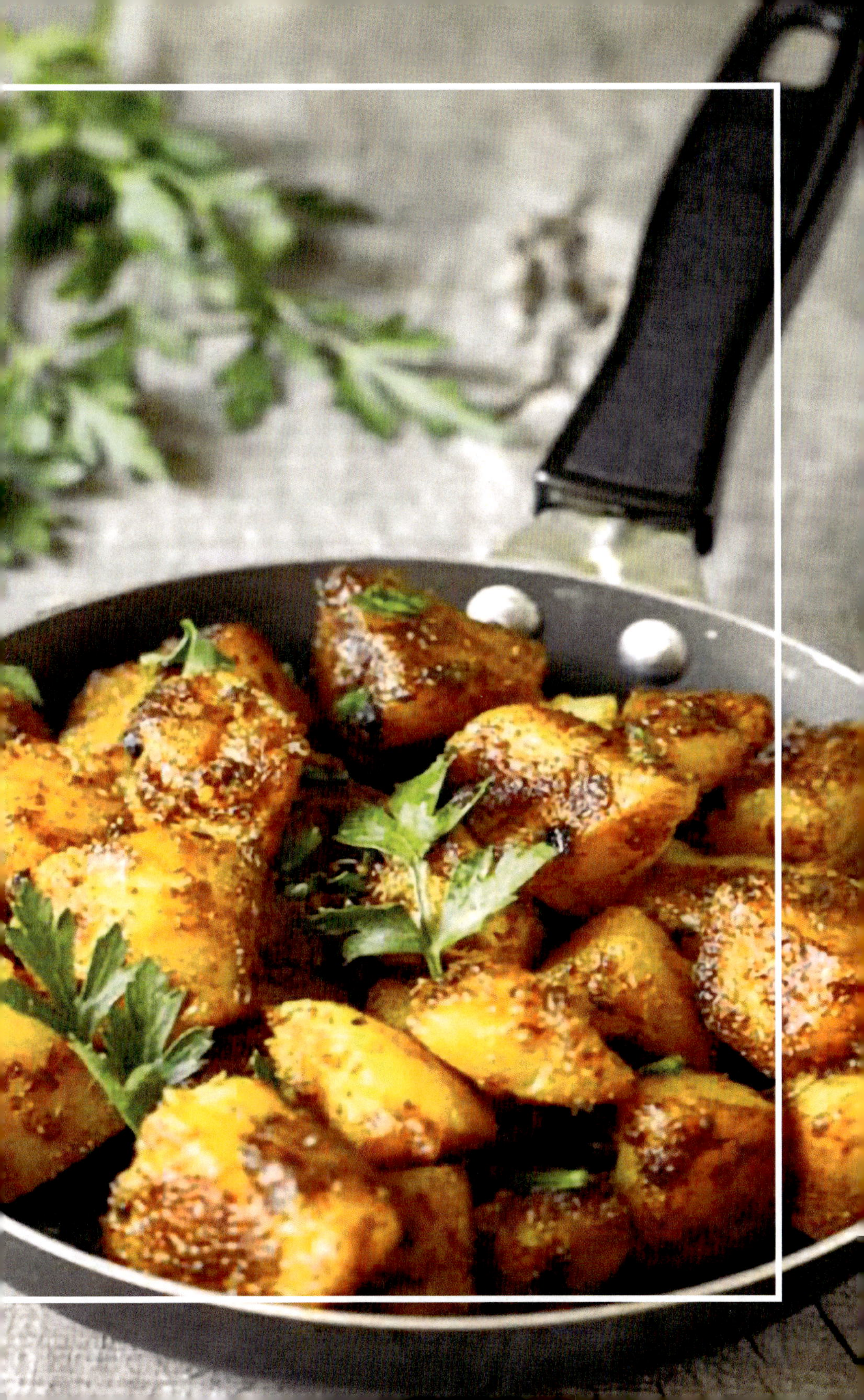

HAITIAN SMOKED HERRING PATTIES

INGREDIENTS

Dough:

2 cups of flour

1 teaspoon of baking powder

½ teaspoon of salt

½ cup + 2 tablespoons of cold water

½ teaspoon of bouillon base or half-crushed bouillon cube

Chicken, Cabbage and Eggs Filling:

1 chicken thigh

½ a lime or lemon, juice reserved

1 tablespoon of epis

1 tablespoon of the reserved liquid from the chicken

¼ teaspoon of salt

⅛ teaspoon of garlic powder

⅛ teaspoon of onion powder

⅛ teaspoon of dried thyme

Pinch of black pepper

1 clove

1 cup of shredded cabbage

1 hard-boiled egg, diced

1 tablespoon of oil

¼ cup of onions, sliced

½ hot pepper, diced (optional)

Hotdogs and Eggs Filling:

1 Hotdog, sliced into 4 strips and diced

1 hard-boiled egg, diced

1 tablespoon of oil

1 tablespoon of epis

¼ cup of onions, sliced

½ hot pepper, diced (optional)

⅛ teaspoon of garlic powder

⅛ teaspoon of onion powder

⅛ teaspoon of dried thyme

Pinch of black pepper

INSTRUCTIONS

Dough:

1. In a small bowl, add water, chicken bouillon base, and mix until the base is dissolved in water.
2. Sift flour into a medium bowl then add baking powder, salt and mix well to combine.
3. Add water mixture to flour using a spoon to mix until a dough forms. Using your hands, begin kneading the dough until it is not sticky, then turn the dough onto the countertop and continue kneading.
4. Form dough into a log, cut in half, then cut each half into 4 pieces to make 8 pieces. Roll each into a ball and using a rolling pin, roll each out, separating them with parchment paper until you're ready to form patties.
5. Herring, Cabbage, and Eggs filling:
6. Bring about 2 cups of water to a boil and set aside. Rub lime half all over the chicken thigh. Pour boiled water over it and let sit for about 30-45 seconds and discard water. Pour the reserved lime juice, clove, and epis over chicken and let marinate for at least an hour.
7. Boil herring in two cups of water for about 25-30 minutes. Once cooked, set aside 1 tablespoon of liquid, remove herring, and allow it to cool. Shred herring and set aside.

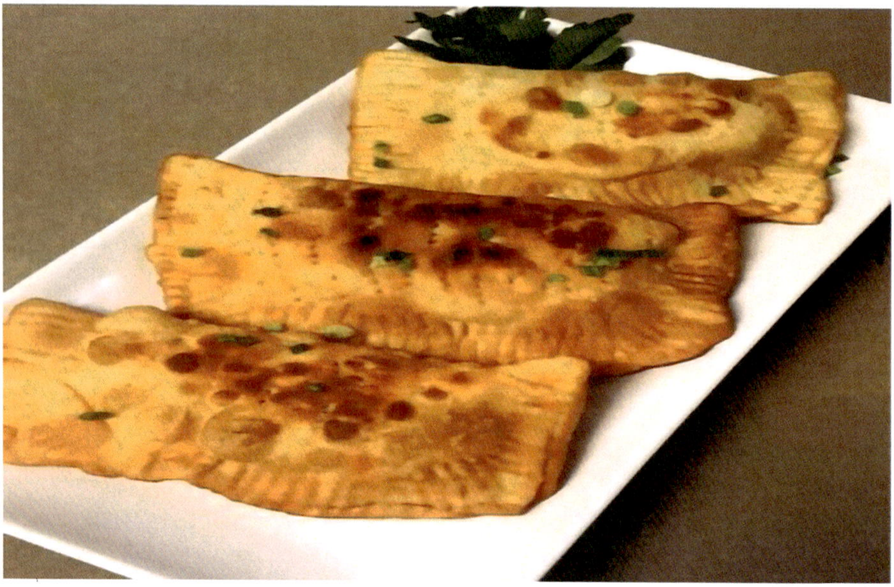

8. On a low to medium heat, add oil to a small skillet, then add herring, sauté for about a minute, then add onions and hot pepper; continue sautéing for 2 minutes.

9. Add dry seasoning, cabbage, reserved liquid, and continue sautéing for another minute. Turn heat off and mix in diced eggs. Pour filling into a bowl and set aside.

10. Add about ⅛ cup filling to half of the rolled-out flour disc, fold the other half over to cover filling, roll edges, or press with a fork to seal the patties.

11. Add about 1-1 ½ cup of oil to the frying pan on a medium to high heat. When the oil is hot, gently place patties in the pan and fry on each side until golden brown. Place on a plate lined with a paper towel and serve while hot!!

12. Hotdogs and Eggs Filling:

13. On low to medium heat, add oil and epis to a small skillet, then add hotdogs, sauté for about a minute, then add onions and hot pepper; continue sautéing for 2 minutes.

14. Add dry seasoning, mix for about a minute, then turn the heat off and mix in diced eggs. Pour filling into a bowl and set aside.

15. Add about 1 ½ tablespoon of filling to half of the rolled-out flour disc, fold the other half over to cover filling roll edges, or press with a fork to seal patties.

16. Add about 1-1 ½ cup of oil to the frying pan on a medium to high heat. When the oil is hot, gently place patties in the pan and fry on each side until golden brown. Place on a plate lined with a paper towel and serve while hot!!

NOTES

1. This recipe will make 4 herring patties and 4 hotdog patties. If you only want to make one, just double your favorite filling recipe to make 8 patties. Once you form your patties, do not, I repeat, do not put them on top of each other, they will stick together, and you will have to rip them when trying to pull them apart. Instead, place them on parchment paper when done forming them.

SHORTCRUST PASTRY, PATE BRISEE

INGREDIENTS

2 cups of flour

1/2 cup of butter or 4oz

1/3 cup of water or 3¼oz

1/4 cup of oil or 2oz

1 teaspoon of salt

1/2 teaspoon of baking powder

12 metal cones

1 clear plastic wrap

INSTRUCTIONS

1. In a cup, mix salt and water together and put aside.
2. On a board, place flour, then create a hole in the center to add butter. Mix it with your hands.
3. Gradually add salted water to the mixture to obtain a soft dough until it doesn't stick to your hands. Bring it into a whole ball.
4. In a clear plastic, brush a little bit of butter, wrap the dough, and let sit for 30 minutes.
5. Flour your board and rolling pin. Roll out the dough to about 1/8 thickness.
6. Brush the metal cone with butter, then cut the flattened dough into 1/2 inch strips to wrap around each cone diagonally starting with the tip.
7. Preheat the oven to 350° F. Place them in a large tray and cook for 20 minutes.
8. Take out the tray and let cool before releasing pastries gently from metal cones.

** You must fill in pastries with a béchamel sauce mixed with sausages or sardines, chunk fish, ham, ground meat, or poultry. Decorate with chopped green and red bell pepper as well as parsley flakes.*

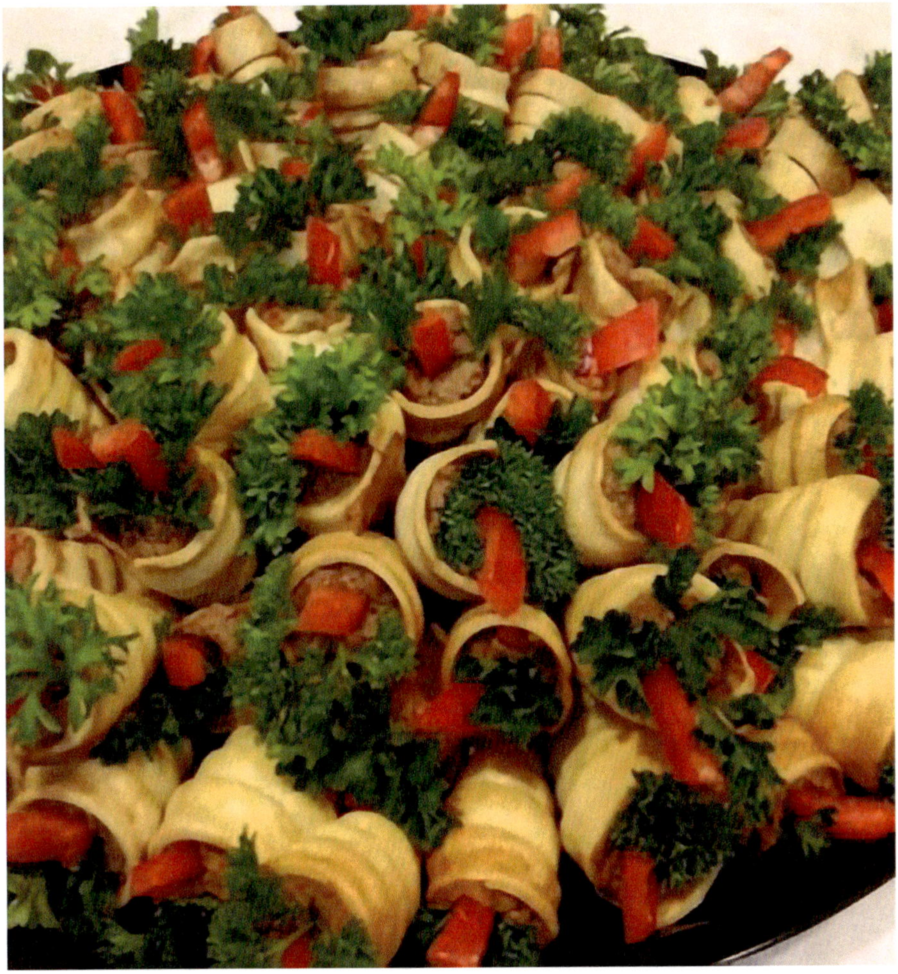

POTATO SCALLOPS

CHEESY GARLIC SCALLOPED POTATOES

Scalloped potatoes are so good, and these cheesy garlic scalloped potatoes are even better. Loaded with three different types of cheese, garlic, and sour cream, these are definitely some tasty taters! Totally scrumptious. A delicious potato casserole that's incredibly satisfying and filling.

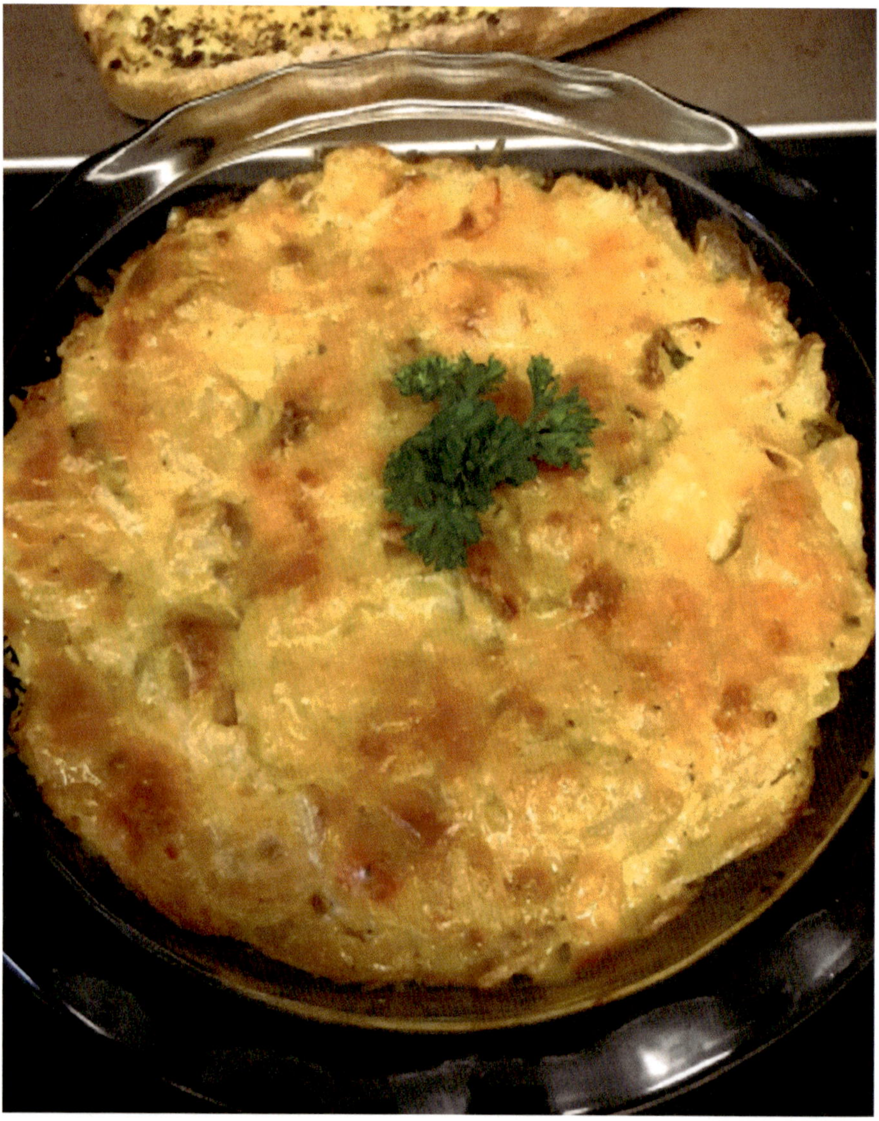

INGREDIENTS

3 tablespoons of butter

1 small white or yellow onion, peeled and thinly sliced

4 large garlic cloves, minced

1/4 cup of all-purpose flour

1 cup of chicken stock or vegetable stock

2 cups of milk (I recommend 2% or whole milk)

1 1/2 teaspoons of Kosher salt

1/2 teaspoon of black pepper

2 teaspoons of fresh thyme leaves, divided

4 pounds of Yukon Gold Potatoes, sliced into 1/8-inch rounds

INSTRUCTIONS

1. Preheat the oven to 400°F. Grease a 9 x 13-inch baking dish with cooking spray; set aside.nnMelt butter in a large sauté pan over medium-high heat. Add onion, and sauté for 4-5 minutes until soft and translucent. Add garlic and sauté for an additional 1-2 minutes until fragrant. Stir in the flour until it is evenly combined, and cook for 1 more minute. Gradually pour in the stock, and whisk until combined. Add in the milk, salt, pepper, and 1 teaspoon of thyme, and whisk until combined. Continue cooking for an additional 1-2 minutes until the sauce just barely begins to simmer around the edges of the pan (avoid letting it come to a boil) and thickens. Then remove from heat and set aside.
2. Spread half of the sliced potatoes in an even layer on the bottom of the pan. Top evenly with half of the cream sauce. (I usually strain out all of the onions and add them here too.) Then sprinkle evenly with 1 cup of the shredded cheddar cheese and all of the Parmesan cheese. Top evenly with the remaining sliced potatoes, the other half of the cream sauce, and the remaining 1 cup of cheddar cheese. Cover the pan with aluminum foil and bake for 30 minutes. The sauce should be nice and bubbly around the edges. Then remove the foil and bake uncovered for 25-30 minutes, or until the potatoes are cooked through. Transfer the pan to a cooling rack, and sprinkle with the remaining teaspoon of thyme and extra Parmesan. Serve warm.
3. 2 cups of freshly-grated sharp cheddar cheese, * divided (feel free to add more cheese if you'd like)
4. 1/2 cup of freshly-grated Parmesan cheese, plus extra for serving

HONEY GARLIC CHICKEN WINGS

INGREDIENTS

Baked Chicken Wings

- 2 lb. chicken wings
- 1 tsp of olive oil
- 1 tsp of sea salt
- 1 pinch of black pepper to taste

Honey Garlic Sauce

- 1/2 cup of honey
- 2 tbsp of soy sauce
- 1 tbsp of fresh ginger grated
- 1 tbsp of garlic minced
- ½ cup of ketchup
- ½ cup of BBQ
- 2 tbsp of hot habanero sauce
- ½ tsp of all-purpose liline creole spices
- ½ tsp of adobo powder
- ½ tsp of garlic powder
- 1/2 tsp of chili powder optional
- fresh cilantro chopped, for garnish (optional)

INSTRUCTIONS

For The Baked Chicken Wings

1. Preheat the oven to 400 degrees F. Line a baking sheet with parchment paper, then set aside.
2. In a large bowl, add raw chicken wings and clean it with lime juice. I usually add some blended creole spice, but you don't have to. But you will definitely have to drizzle with olive oil and season with salt and pepper and all-purpose liline creole spices. Use a pair of tongs or a spatula to gently toss the chicken wings to coat.
3. Arrange chicken wings in an even layer on the prepared baking sheet.
4. Bake chicken wings for 40 minutes or until juices run clear, turning them halfway through.

For The Honey Garlic Sauce

1. In a medium saucepan over medium-high heat, bring honey, soy sauce, ketchup, BBQ, habanero, ginger, garlic, adobo, and chili powder (optional) to a rapid boil. Allow to simmer, occasionally stirring for 3-4 minutes or until sauce is reduced by 1/2.
2. Remove saucepan from heat. Cover and set aside.

Putting It All Together

1. Working quickly, place baked chicken wings in a bowl, then pour prepared honey garlic glaze on top. This step works best if both the chicken and the sauce are hot. Use a spatula to toss the chicken wings until they are coated in the glaze. Note: It's okay if the glaze is thick, but it should pour easily. If it doesn't, microwave the glaze for 30 seconds at a time until it's liquid again, then quickly pour over the chicken wings.
2. Serve honey garlic chicken wings immediately with chopped cilantro as garnish (optional).

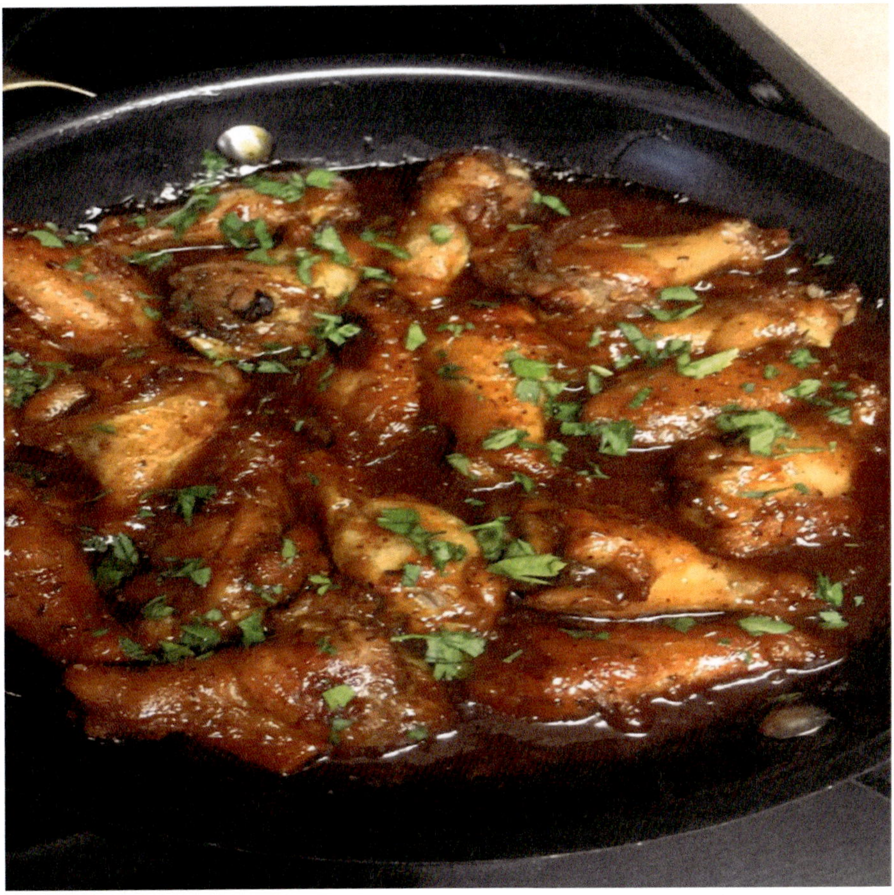

BOMBAY POTATOES RECIPES INDIAN FOOD

INGREDIENTS

12 tsp of cumin of potato cubes	1/4 tsp of turmeric powder, optional
3 tbsp of oil	1½ tsp of lemon juice
2 tsp of green chili paste	Salt to taste

INSTRUCTIONS

1. Heat the oil in a non-stick skillet and add the cumin seeds.
2. When the seeds crackle, add the potatoes, mix well, cover with a lid and cook on a medium flame for 10 to 12 minutes or till the potatoes are cooked, while stirring occasionally.
3. Add the green chili paste, turmeric powder, lemon juice, salt, and cilantro, mix well and cook on a medium flame for a minute or two, again stirring occasionally.
4. Serve hot.

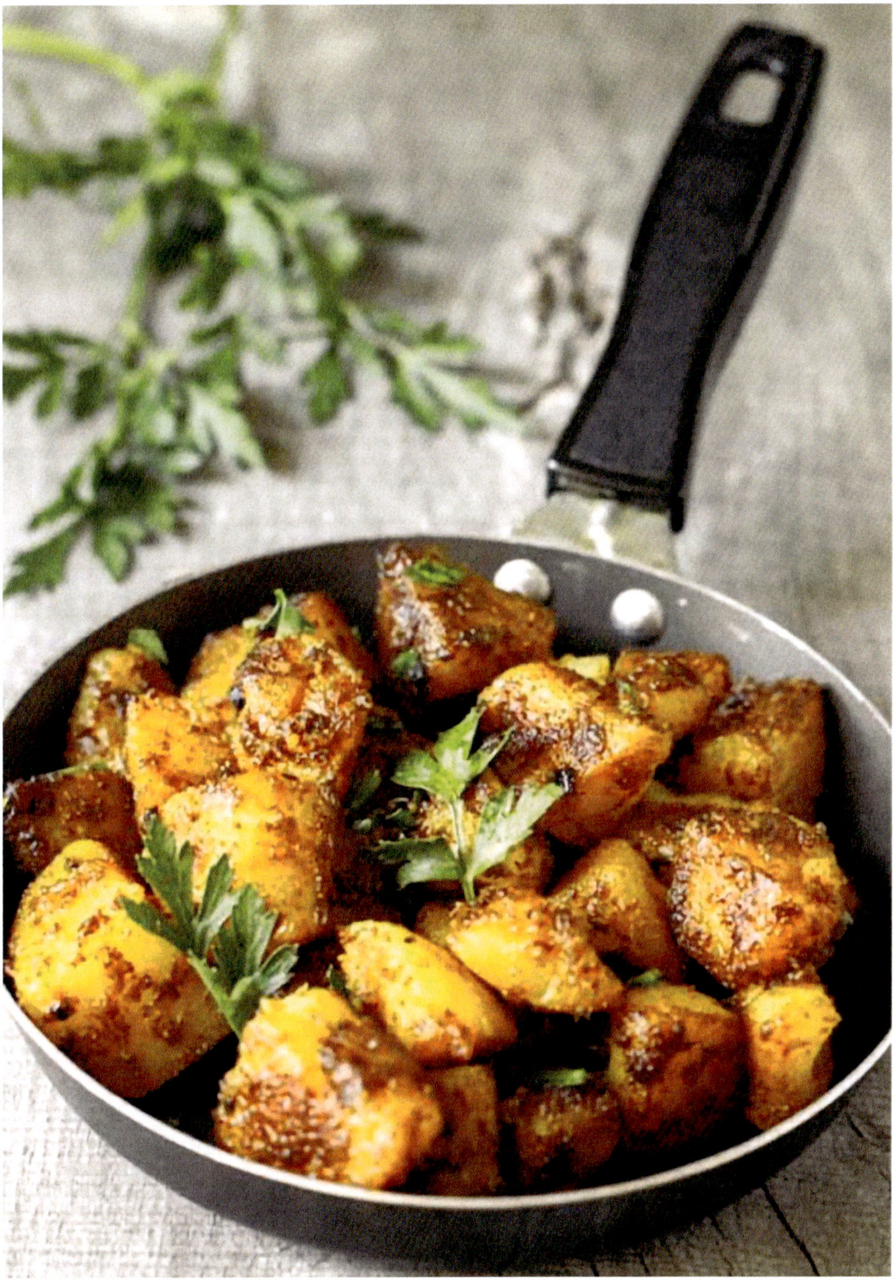

NEW ORLEANS JAMBALAYA RECIPE

Jambalaya is one of Louisiana's most famous dishes that has both French and Spanish influence. It's quite similar in style to Spanish Paella in that it has rice and often seafood. Cajun Style Jambalaya tends to be browner in color as the meat is cooked first in the pot, then the vegetables are sautéed after that and cooked in the rice with stock.

Creole style, also known as 'red jambalaya,' includes tomatoes, which are cooked along with the trinity of vegetables, onions, bell peppers, and celery, and then cooked with the rice and stock as before.

INGREDIENTS

Meat

2 chicken breasts, boneless skinless

1 (14-ounces) of package Eckrich smoked sausage

Produce

3 Bell peppers, small

2 Celery, ribs of

4 cloves of Garlic

1/2 tsp of Garlic powder

1 Jalapeno

1 1/4 cup of Okra

1/2 tsp of onion powder

1 tsp of Oregano, dried

1 Red onion, medium

1/4 tsp of Thyme, dried

1 (28-ounces) of can Tomatoes

Canned Goods

3 cups of Chicken broth

Pasta & Grains

2 cups of Rice, long-grain

Baking & Spices

1 tsp of Black pepper

1 Cajun spice blend, Homemade

1 tsp of Cayenne pepper

1 tsp of Paprika

1 Salt and pepper

1 1/2 tsp of Sea salt

Oils & Vinegars

4 tbsp of Olive oil

Other

1 pound of raw shrimp, deveined and tail removed

INSTRUCTIONS

1. In a large heavy pan with a lid, add two tablespoons of olive oil. Add in the celery, bell pepper, onion, jalapeno, and garlic. Sauté the veggies over medium-high heat until they begin to get tender. On my gas stovetop, this takes about four minutes.
2. Sprinkle the chicken pieces with salt and pepper. Add another two tablespoons of olive oil to the pan with the veggies. Fold in the chicken and Eckrich Smoked Sausage. Continue to sauté everything until the chicken is almost cooked and no longer pink.
3. Add in the chicken broth, crushed tomatoes, rice, and homemade Cajun seasoning blend. Mix with a wooden spoon to combine all ingredients. Add two bay leaves. Cover the pan with a lid and lower the heat to medium-low. Allow the jambalaya to simmer until the rice is fully cooked and tender. On my stovetop, this takes 25 minutes. While the jambalaya is simmering, stir the ingredients every 4-5 minutes to prevent the rice from sticking to the bottom of the pan and burning.
4. Fold in the shrimp and okra. Cover the pan again and allow the shrimp to cook until done. Once done, remove the two bay leaves from the pot. Do a taste test and see if you need to add in some additional salt and pepper or slightly increase the heat with a sprinkling of more cayenne pepper.
5. Your delicious jambalaya is ready to be garnished with green onions and fresh parsley leaves.

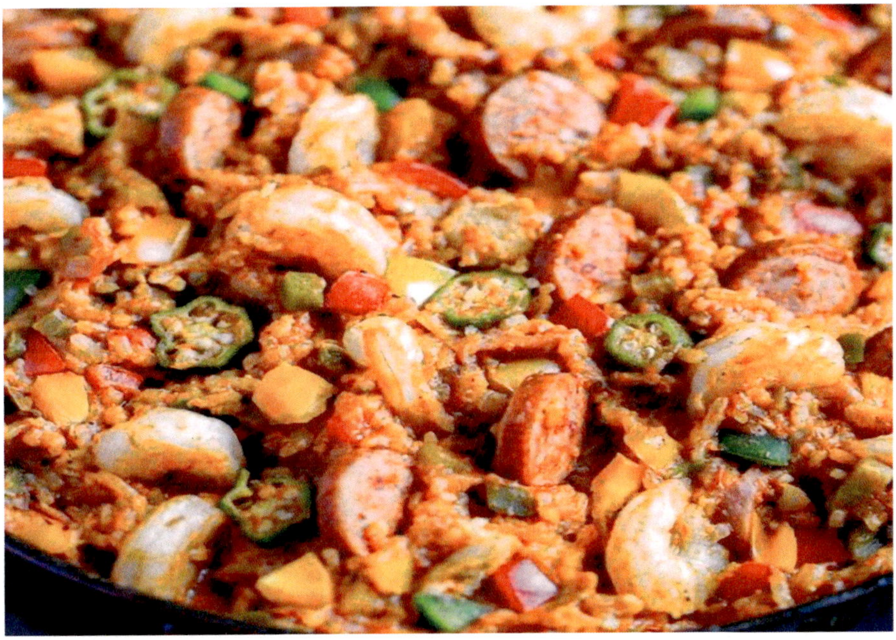

BLACK RICE/ MUSHROOM RICE

WHAT IS DJON DJON (BLACK MUSHROOM)

This particular mushroom is found all over Haiti, particularly in the northern region of Haiti. It is known as a delicacy and is often served at weddings, holidays, Sunday dinners, or on special occasions.

HOW TO PREPARE DJON DJON

It is best to soak the mushroom overnight for intense flavor, but it can be boiled prior to cooking in order to retrieve the water. Though the boiling process may be quicker and more convenient, personally, I think it uses more djon djon than necessary.

However, I have blended it sometimes, which I especially like since it uses the entire djon djon, and nothing is lost. It is especially helpful if you are pressed for time, as it will extract the dark color of the djon djon directly to prepare the rice.

If you so choose to do the overnight or the boiling process, the black mushroom/djon djon is to be discarded after the water has been extracted from it. Unlike other mushrooms that are visible in the dishes, such as this mushroom soup, you will not see the mushroom in the rice.

HOW TO MAKE HAITIAN BLACK RICE – DIRI DJON DJON

As mentioned above, there are a few methods to use to make Haitian black rice. For this recipe, the actual mushroom is not easily available in my region. Therefore, traveling to areas that are populated with Haitians isn't always possible. For this reason, I used the Maggi Djon Djon.

INGREDIENTS

- 2 cups of long-grain rice
- 3 cups of dried black mushrooms
- 12 oz pre-cooked shrimp (skinless)
- 1/4 chopped green & red bell pepper
- 2 garlic cloves crushed
- 1/4 cup of chopped onion and parsley
- 1 scotch bonnet pepper
- 1 cup of frozen Lima beans or green peas
- 3 tablespoons of olive oil or vegetable oil
- 6 cloves & 2 thyme sprigs
- 2 teaspoons of salt
- 2 teaspoons of lime juice
- 6 cups of water
- 1/4 crushed scallion

INSTRUCTIONS

1. Clean and boil black mushrooms in 4 cups of water (10 minutes).
2. In another saucepan, bring to a boil 2 cups of water, pour over pre-cooked shrimp, let sit 2 minutes, remove shrimp from hot water, and season with lime juice and ground pices.
3. Sautee skinless shrimp in 1 tablespoon of oil on medium heat until tender and put aside.
4. In a cast-iron pot, sauté onions in 2 tablespoons of oil, green & red bell pepper, green or Lima beans, crushed garlic, scallion, and stir up to 5 minutes on medium heat. When done, save half of cooked spices and beans for later. In a large pot, add your djon-djon and 8-10 cups of water and bring it to a boil. Once boiled, use a strainer to drain and set the liquid aside.
5. Add strained mushroom water in a pot along with cloves, scotch bonnet pepper, parsley, thyme, salt, and also 6 to 8 sautéed shrimp.
6. Bring water to a boil, taste it for the desired flavor, then rinse the rice with cold water and add into boiling water.
7. Let simmer until water evaporates, then spread the saved portion of Lima beans or green peas as well as remaining sautéed shrimp over rice. Make sure scotch bonnet pepper stayed on top before stirring the rice.
8. Lower heat, cover the rice and let cook for 20 to 25 minutes.
9. Before serving, remove scotch bonnet pepper, stir the rice with remaining sautéed shrimp, and Bon Appétit!

ARROZ CON GANDULES/ PUERTO RICO

Arroz con Gandules is one of Puerto Rico's iconic rice dishes. Whether served simply with pollo, or stuffed inside a lechon, or roasted pig, soaking in bubbling pig fat, this rich, rice recipe is one that every household in Puerto Rico has a variation on

INGREDIENTS

- 3 cups of medium-grain rice
- 3 cups of water
- 1 can of gandules (pigeon peas) drained
- 1/2 cup of cured salted pork chopped
- 1/3 cup of vegetable oil
- 1/2 cup of sofrito
- 6 oz tomato sauce
- 1 packet of sazon culantro y achiote
- 10 whole Spanish olives
- 1 tsp of cumin
- salt for taste

INSTRUCTIONS

1. Start by adding the vegetable oil to the caldero or a large pot, and set the stove heat to medium. Toss in your chopped cured salted pork into the pot and cook until it is fried. Remove the cured salted pork and set aside but keep the grease in the caldero.
2. Next, add your sofrito, tomato sauce, sazon culantro y achiote, cumin, Spanish olives, and gandules to the caldero. Cook and stir the mixture for about 3 to 4 minutes. In addition, add your water and bring to a boil. Rinse your medium-grain rice to remove starch.
3. Lastly, add your medium grain rice and the fried cured salted pork and stir everything gently. Place a sheet of foil covering the top opening of the caldero and cover it with a lid. Cook the Puerto Rican rice for 30 minutes over medium heat without opening the lid at all. Fluff rice and add salt for personal taste.

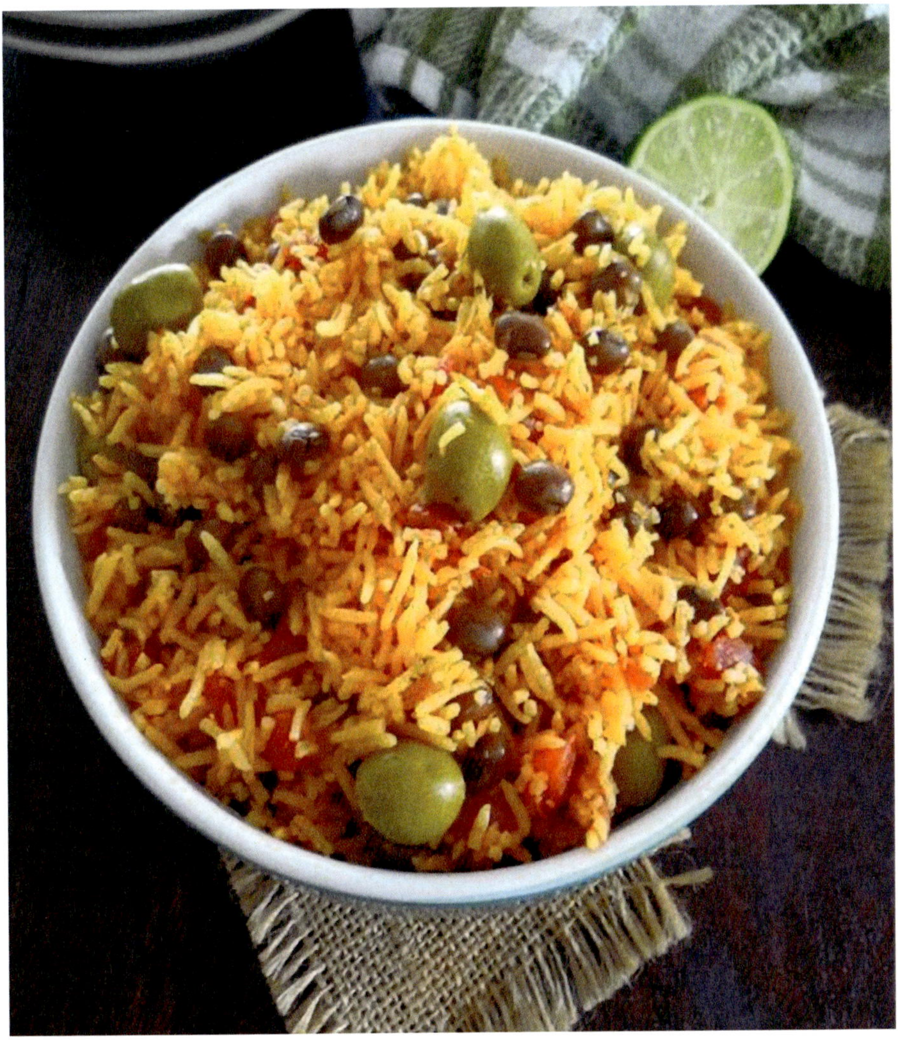

RECIPE NOTES

1. *For a perfect water amount, make sure the rice is below liquid by 1 inch before placing the foil and caldero lid.*
2. *Do not wash the starch off of the rice if you prefer your rice sticky.*

BRAISED CHICKEN FEET

In the foodie's recipes, the chicken feet are called the Phoenix foot. In the south, the chicken feet are a top-grade dish, and the cooking method is more complicated. With the variety of cooking methods, this variety of dishes is popular in China.

INGREDIENTS

- 750g chicken feet
- 2 teaspoons of light soy sauce
- 1 tablespoon of ginger, minced
- 3 tablespoons of dark soy sauce
- 1/2 teaspoon of salt
- 1 tablespoon of cooking wine
- 2 star anises
- 2 small cinnamons
- 2 fragrant leaves
- 1 teaspoon of Sichuan peppercorns, black seeds removed then ground
- 10g rock sugar
- 1/2 teaspoon of the thirteen kinds of spices

INSTRUCTIONS

1. Cut the claws off and any dirty part on the chicken feet. Then wash it several times and then soak in the water for half an hour.
2. Bring enough water in a wok, add the chicken feet and cook it under high heat until boiling. Continue to cook for 3 minutes. Dump water and transfer chicken feet in a basin, and then rinse with running water and drain completely.
3. Pour the chicken feet and the clean water just enough to cover the chicken feet in a wok and cook until boiling.
4. Add ginger, light soy sauce, dark soy sauce, and cooking wine in the wok and mix well.
5. Add anise, fragrant leaves, cinnamon, Sichuan peppercorns, rock sugar, and the thirteen kinds of spices in the wok. Cook it until boiling. Reduce the fire and continue to cook for 80 minutes. Then cook it under high heat until the sauce has thickened. Transfer it on a plate. Serve.

Notes

1. **Cleaning:** The chicken feet have a smell of earthworm and need to be rinsed. However, during the rinsing process, it is important to remove the small yellow sputum from the palm and remove the yellow "coat" remaining on the chicken claws. Cut the claws off and any dirty part on the chicken feet. This is very important! Rinsing the chicken feet and soaked them. When soaking, it is best to put it in the water with some onion, ginger, and cooking wine, soak it for 3~4 hours. Bring enough water in a wok, add the chicken feet and cook it under high heat until boiling. Continue to cook for 3 minutes. Dump water and transfer chicken feet in a basin, and then rinse with running water and drain completely.

2. Since soy sauce is salty, you can choose whether to add salt or not.

3. The taste of the chicken feet can be adjusted according to your preference. If you like to eat chewy, cook it for a short time.

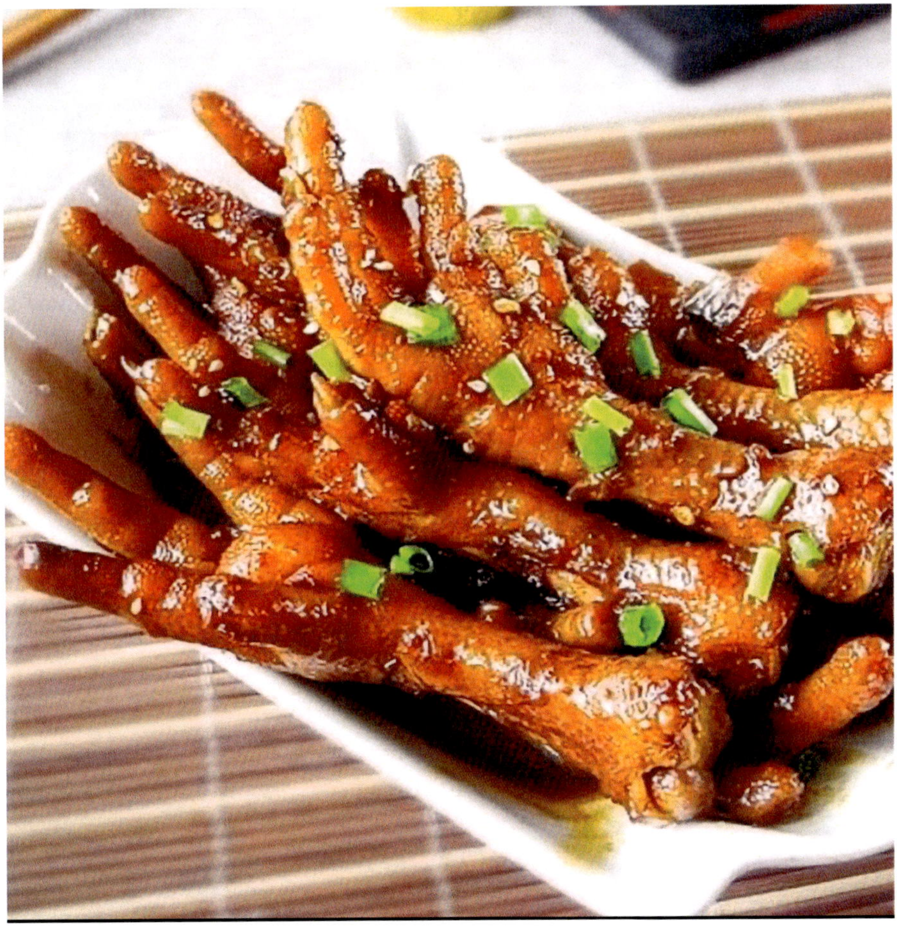

SWEET PLANTAINS LASAGNA

There are a lot of dishes that make me think of home, but there is no doubt that my favorite is Pastelon. It's one of those dishes that I don't get to enjoy often, so when I do, it's a real treat. If you're not familiar with pastelon, your life is incomplete. It's basically a lasagna, but, in my opinion, better in place of noodles, you use sweet fried plantains.

INGREDIENTS

Meat

1 lbs. of Ground beef

Produce

2 Bay leaves

1/2 Cilantro bunch

3 cloves of Garlic

1 Green pepper

1 Onion

tsp of Oregano

4 Plantains, ripe

1/2 cup of Raisins

Refrigerated

3 Eggs

Canned Goods

2 tsp of Adobo

Condiments

8 Stuffed olives, green

1/4 cup of Tomato sauce

Baking & Spices

1 Salt

Oils & Vinegars

1 Vegetable oil

2 tbsp of Vinegar

Dairy

2 cups of Cheese, white

2 tbsp of Milk

Other

1 envelope Salón

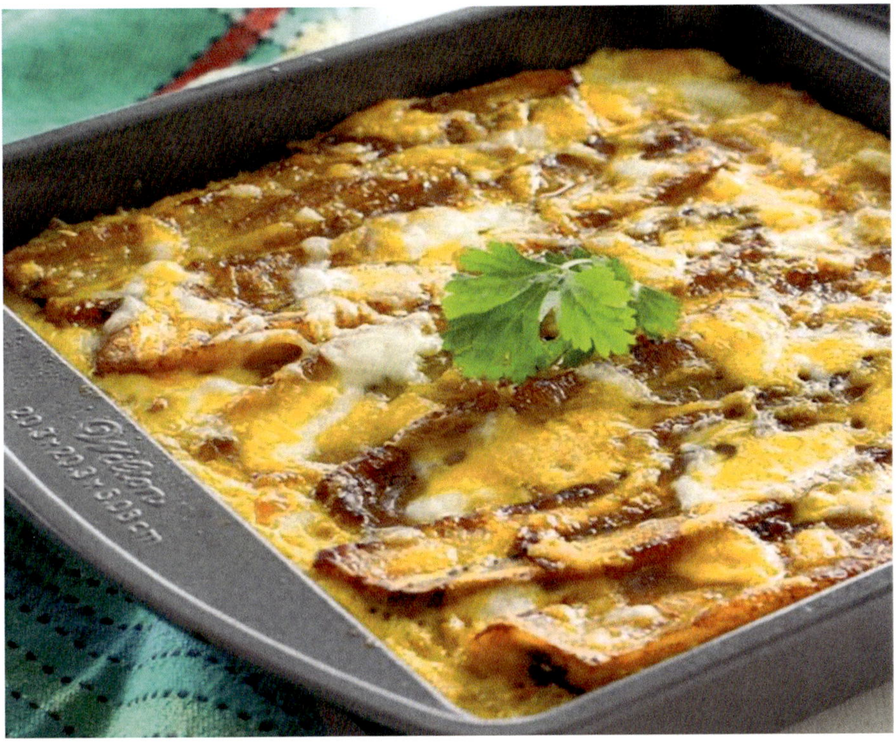

INSTRUCTIONS

1. Preheat the oven to 350 degrees. Butter square pan with 1 tbsp of butter.
2. Combine beef, onion, pepper, garlic, cilantro, adobo, oregano, vinegar, and sazon. Mix well.
3. Heat a large skillet over medium-high heat with 2 Tbsp of olive oil, add meat mixture.
4. Cook beef until brown, and if the juices bubble up, add bay leaves, olives, raisins, and tomato sauce. Mix and let simmer for 10 minutes, set aside.
5. Heat a large frying pan with vegetable oil, just enough to coat the bottom. Fry plantains for 2-3 minutes on each side or until golden and slightly crispy. Drain on a plate with a paper towel, set aside.
6. To assemble pastelon: Take your prepared square pan, start with a layer of plantains, then beef, then a fistful of cheese, repeat. You want to finish with cheese and plantains. Beat 3 eggs with 2 Tbsp of milk, pour over the pastelón. Let it sit for a minute allowing the egg to soak in. Top off with just a bit more cheese.
7. Bake in the oven at 350 degrees for 20 minutes.

CARIBBEAN CHICKEN ROTI RECIPE

Chicken Roti is a fantastic street food dish served in many parts of the Caribbean. This chicken recipe covers both the filling and the roti flatbread, but you can, of course, just opt for the filling and buy the bread from your favorite supplier or supermarket.

This delicious recipe comes courtesy of Tan Rosie Foods and originates from India via Trinidad.

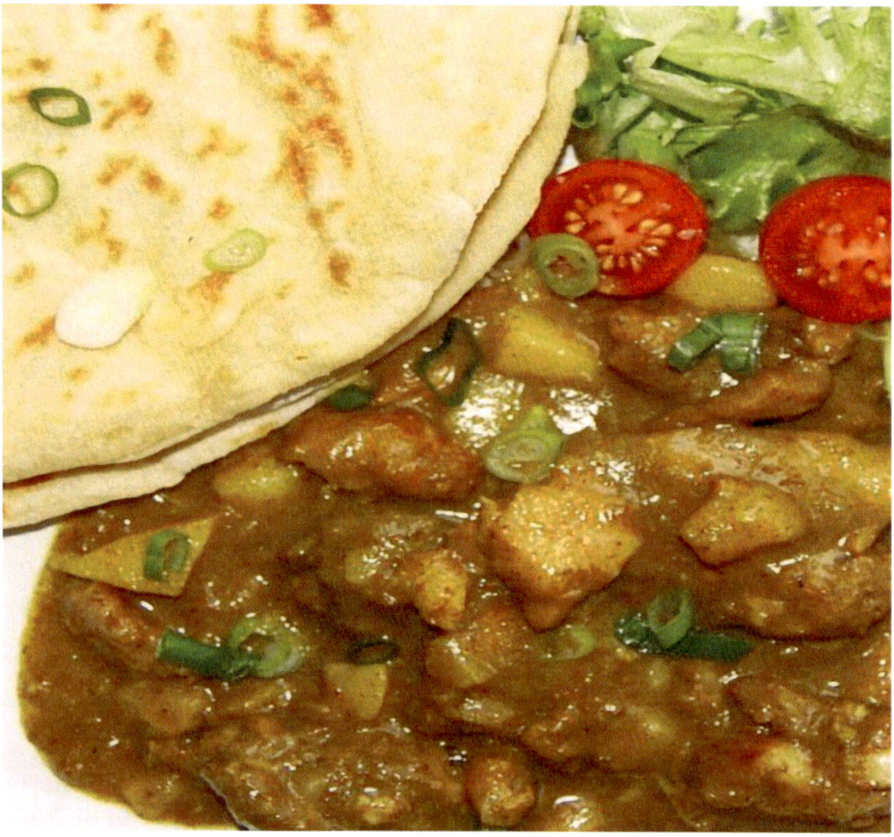

Tip:

Make sure you have a plate and warm towel ready for the rotis. Plus, it's important to leave the chicken to marinate for at least 2 hours or overnight.

INGREDIENTS

500gm Boned Chicken Thighs (Cubed).

40gm Tan Rosie Caribbean Style Curry Powder

1 tbsp of Vegetable Oil

1 Scotch Bonnet Pepper

1 medium Potato (Cubed)

200ml Coconut Milk

1 Large Onion (Minced)

2 Garlic Cloves (Minced)

1 tsp of Salt & Black Pepper

100 ml Water

Roti Ingredients

500gm of Flour

1 tbsp of Baking Powder

1 tsp of Salt

50gm Ghee

Water enough to form a soft dough

INSTRUCTIONS

To make the Chicken Curry:

1. Cut boned chicken thigh into cubes.
2. Massage curry powder into chicken & leave overnight.
3. Heat oil in a pan, then add onions & sauté for 5mins until golden brown.
4. Add minced garlic & sauté for 1 minute.
5. Add the seasoned chicken and fry until brown.
6. Add coconut milk, water, potato, salt, pepper & scotch bonnet pepper, and cover pot and bring to boil & simmer for 40mins.
7. Remove cover and reduce liquid until thickened.
8. Remove scotch bonnet pepper and serve.

To Make Roti:

1. Add flour, salt & baking powder into a bowl.
2. Add some water (enough to form a soft, pliable dough) then mix for 5 mins.
3. Turn out onto the floured surface & knead until smooth – cover & leave for 15mins.
4. Melt ghee in a pan and add some flour to make a paste, then cut dough into 4 portions and make round balls and roll out into 10" disc.
5. Brush ghee paste onto the disc and cut from the center of the disc to the outer edge and roll together to form a cone shape.
6. Place the cone on the surface, push the peak down, so it is flat and roll out into a 12" diameter disc (the cone shape makes the layers).
7. Place on a hot tawa or girdle stone and cook for 1 min – turn and brush with ghee and repeat until brown spots appear.
8. Remove and cover with a warm towel – then repeat until all the dough is cooked.

JAMAICAN JERK CHICKEN DRUMSTICKS WITH BROWN RICE

The flavors of Jamaica in your own home! These chicken drumsticks have a really punchy, strong flavor. Make them as spicy as you want - or not! These are really tasty even if you pull back - or even leave out - the chili. This recipe is adapted from Oven Baked Jerk Chicken recipe

INGREDIENTS

8 (about 2.5lb / 1.2kg) chicken drumsticks (Note 1)

Marinade

2 tbsp of olive oil

1 tbsp of soy sauce

1 lime (or 1/2 lemon), juice only (about 2 tbsp)

1 onion, coarsely chopped (brown, yellow, or white)

1 tbsp of fresh ginger, chopped (or 1 tsp of dried ginger powder)

1 or more scotch bonnet pepper or substitute with another chili (Note 2)

6 garlic cloves, roughly chopped

2 tsp of salt

2 tsp of black pepper

3 tbsp of brown sugar

1/2 tbsp of cinnamon powder

1/2 tbsp of allspice powder

1/2 tsp of nutmeg powder (preferably freshly grated)

1/2 tsp of dried thyme or 1 sprig of fresh thyme

Garnish

Fresh cilantro/coriander leaves

INSTRUCTIONS

1. Pat the chicken dry with a paper towel and place in a large zip lock bag.
2. Place Marinade ingredients in a food processor and whizz until smooth. Try not to touch the Marinade with bare hands to avoid getting chili on your hands.
3. Pour the Marinade into the zip lock bag. Close the bag, squeezing out excess air. Massage the bag from the outside to disperse the Marinade throughout the chicken. Marinate for at least 4 hours or up to 24 hours.
4. When ready to cook, remove the chicken from the marinade, but reserve the Marinade.

Oven

1. Preheat the oven to 180C/350
2. Place a wire rack on a baking tray lined with foil. Place the drumsticks on the rack and baste the top with half the Marinade. Bake for 25 minutes.
3. Turn the drumsticks and baste the top with the remaining Marinade. Bake for a further 20 to 25 minutes, until the drumsticks are very dark brown.
4. Rest for 5 minutes before serving, garnished with coriander/cilantro if using.

Bbq/Grill

1. Preheat the grill side of the BBQ on medium
2. Brush the grill with oil, if required.
3. Place the chicken on the grill. Brush the top with 1/2 the Marinade. Cook for 10 minutes, then turn.
4. Brush the top with the remaining Marinade and cook for a further 5 to 8 minutes.
5. Then turn the chicken again (to cook the side that you just brushed Marinade on) and cook for a few minutes. Total cook time around 20 minutes in total.
6. Remove from the BBQ and rest for 5 minutes before serving, garnished with coriander/cilantro if using.

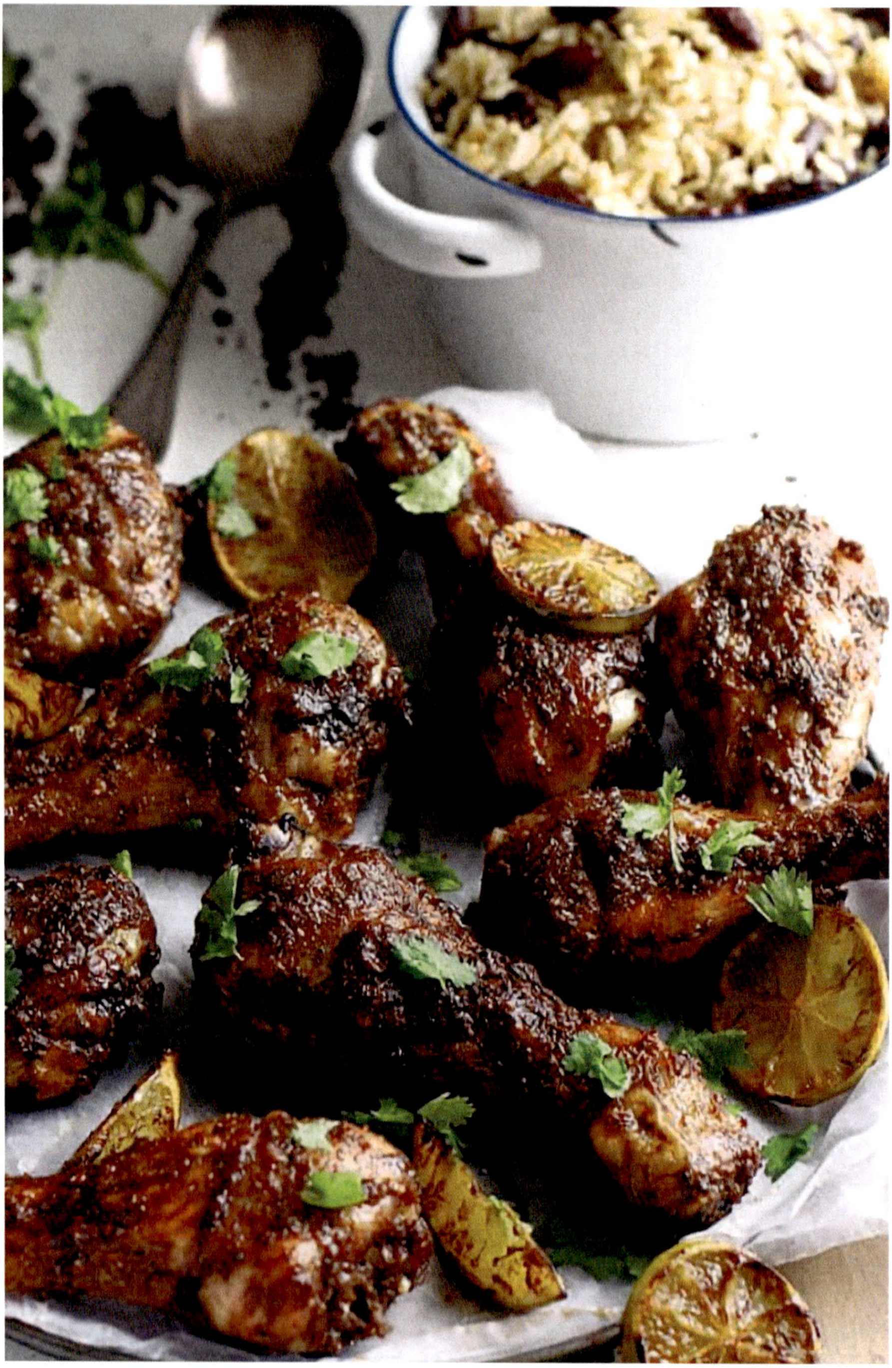

Recipe Notes:

1. *This recipe works really well with chicken thigh fillets with or without skin, with or without bone. It works, but it is not as good with chicken breast. You really need fat for the Marinade to mix with and to caramelize. If you use boneless chicken thigh fillets, you can also cook this on the stove.*

2. *The original recipe calls for 1+ scotch bonnet peppers (adjust according to taste). Scotch bonnet peppers are a very hot chili that are commonly used in African and Caribbean cooking. On the chili "heat" scale, it is about 50% spicier than the bird's eye chili. The best substitute is habanero peppers, which is about the same level of spiciness. Otherwise, a bird's eyes or any other spicy chili is an adequate substitute. Just do a taste test of the marinade to get the spiciness to your taste. You can get dried habaneros in Australia from Herbies or Fireworks Food. Just soak in a bit of warm water for 15 minutes or so, then put it straight into the food processor without sautéing. I find 2 habaneros / 3 bird's eye chilies to give it a nice kick. If I'm cooking for someone who can't handle spicy food, I reduce it to 1 bird's eye chili. If you are using a scotch bonnet or habanero peppers, be aware that they are very hot! Use gloves if you can, and wash your hands, food processor, and anything else that has come into contact with them. DO NOT rub your eyes!! Or any other sensitive part of your body!*

3. *The original recipe calls for using the Marinade to make a sauce by simmering it on the stove for 7 minutes with the juices from the chicken. I changed it to use all the Marinade on the chicken, so the drumsticks are coated with a thicker flavor, rather than sauce on the side. The other reason I did this is that drumsticks in Australia don't drop enough juice and fat to be able to create enough liquid to turn the remaining Marinade into a sauce. Also, I like the thicker, stronger flavor on the chicken.*

4. *Jerk Chicken goes fabulously with Caribbean Rice and Beans (see recipe below).*

5. *Nutrition for the Jamaican Jerk Chicken Drumsticks based on 4 servings.*

LALO WITH BEEF AND SEAFOOD, SPINACH

Lalo (jute leaves) is a leaf packed with minerals, vitamins, and antioxidants that has an intense green color; it is slightly rough yet a little slimy kind of texture. It is the beloved signature dish of Latibonit (Artibonite), but a lot of people in other regions of Haiti cook this dish, not only Latibonit people.

Jute leaves are very nutritious, rich in calcium, iron, protein, vitamin A, C, and E, thiamin, riboflavin, niacin, folate, and dietary fibers. Jute leaves are found in specialty stores fresh, frozen or dried form. It can also be found at local farmers' markets, depending on your location, and it may be called okra leaves. Not the same leaves from the okra plant.

INGREDIENTS

For the beef

- 2 pounds of stew beef
- 1 lime or lemon to clean the meat
- 3 garlic cloves chopped finely
- 1 small white onion chopped
- 1 sprig of thyme
- 2 scallions chopped finely
- 2 tablespoons of parsley chopped finely
- ½ lime juice
- ½ teaspoon of salt
- Black pepper to taste
- 1/8 teaspoon of ground cloves
- 1 tablespoon of chicken bouillon or beef bouillon cube
- 2 tablespoon of olive oil
- 2 tablespoons of tomato paste
- ½ teaspoon of hot sauce or ½ hot pepper

For the Lalo or Jute Leaves

- 4 cups of dried Lalo or Jute leaves
- 8 cups of water
- 1 pinch of baking soda
- Soak 30 minutes

For the Spinach

12 ounces bag of baby spinach or regular spinach

Clean roughly chopped and set aside

For the Blue Crabs

2 – 4 blue crabs

1 lemon

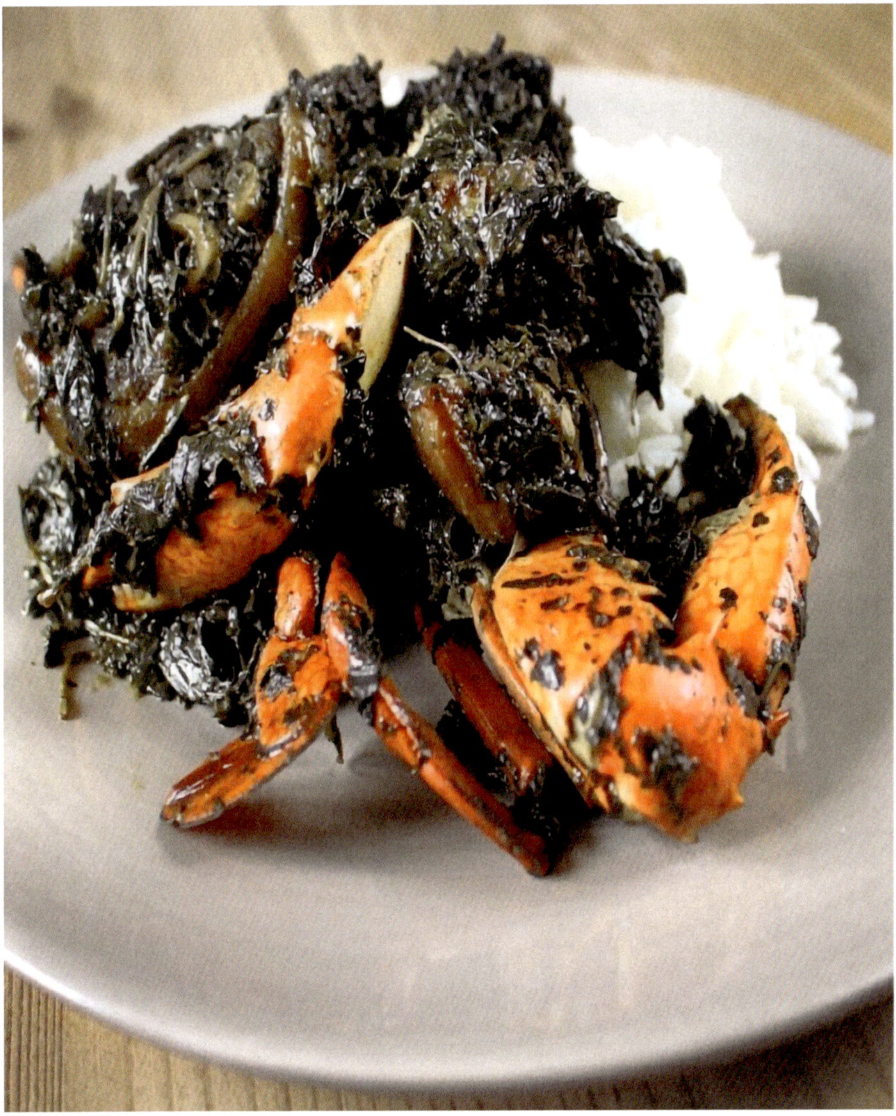

INSTRUCTIONS

Thoroughly clean crabs with lemon or lime. Please see this link on how to clean crab http://www.bluecrab.info/cbyc.html. Reserve shells if you prefer. Add to a bowl and add salt and pepper to taste with a little bit of lemon juice. Refrigerate until use.

1. Remove dried Lalo or Jute leaves from packaging and remove any debris. Place in a large bowl and add water with baking soda. Let soak for 30 minutes.
2. To marinate beef: In a bowl, place beef pieces and clean with lemon or vinegar. Rinse under cool water and pat dry. In a clean bowl, add lemon or lime juice, garlic, onion, thyme, scallions, parsley, salt, black pepper, ground cloves, chicken bouillon, or beef bouillon and let marinate for at least 30 minutes.
3. Strain Lalo and discard water and set aside
4. In a heavy bottom pan, heat oil and add tomato paste. Fry for about 1 – 2 minutes. Add beef and marinade and stir to mix. Add hot pepper or hot sauce—lower heat.
5. Add Lalo or Jute leaves to cover the meat.

Add spinach

Cover with aluminum foil

Cover the pot with a fitted lid and let cook until beef is cooked thoroughly, for about 40 – 55 minutes.

1. Remove aluminum foil and add clean blue crabs to the mixture and stir to incorporate.
2. Cook uncovered until crabs are cooked, about 15 to 20 minutes.
3. Remove from the stovetop, remove hot pepper and serve immediately with rice or root vegetables

NOTES

Add baking soda to dried jute leaves (lalo) to slow down the sliminess process.

Lalo can be cooked with seafood (crab, conch, or shrimp) only, and not with red meat if preferred. Cooking time will differ depending on the seafood.

Always use a wooden spoon when making this dish. That will allow the leaves to cook well and the texture of the dish to be correct and the dish to be appetizing.

FIRECRACKER SALMON RECIPE

INGREDIENTS

- 1 teaspoon of minced garlic
- 1/2 teaspoon of minced ginger
- 1 tablespoon of olive oil
- 1 tablespoon of low sodium low soy sauce
- 2 tablespoons of Heinz chili sauce (substitute with Buffalo sauce or hot sauce to suit your heat preference)
- 1 teaspoon of brown sugar (or brown sugar substitute) -- OPTIONAL
- pinch of crushed red chili flakes
- 1-2 teaspoons of sriracha (adjust to suit your heat preference)
- 4 skin of salmon fillets
- Salt and pepper to season
- 1/2 teaspoon of paprika (mild, smoky, or spicy)
- 1/4 cup of chives chopped

INSTRUCTIONS

1. In a shallow bowl, whisk together the minced garlic, minced ginger, olive oil, soy sauce, chili sauce, brown sugar, red chili flakes, and sriracha to combine.
2. Season salmon with salt, pepper, and paprika. Add salmon fillets to the marinade, turning each to evenly coat in the sauce.
3. Cover with plastic wrap and let marinate in the refrigerator for 2 hours or overnight (if time allows).
4. Preheat the oven to 370°F (190°C). Heat an oven-proof skillet over medium heat with a small drizzle of oil.
5. Sear salmon for 2-3 minutes on both sides, undisturbed, to get a nice crust. (You may need to sear in batches depending on the size of your skillet.)
6. Transfer to a plate and repeat with remaining salmon.
7. Return all salmon fillets to the skillet. Alternatively, transfer to a baking dish.
8. Bake for 8-10 minutes, or until cooked to your liking.
9. Serve warm with chopped chives.

05
SIDES THAT GO WITH ANY MEAL

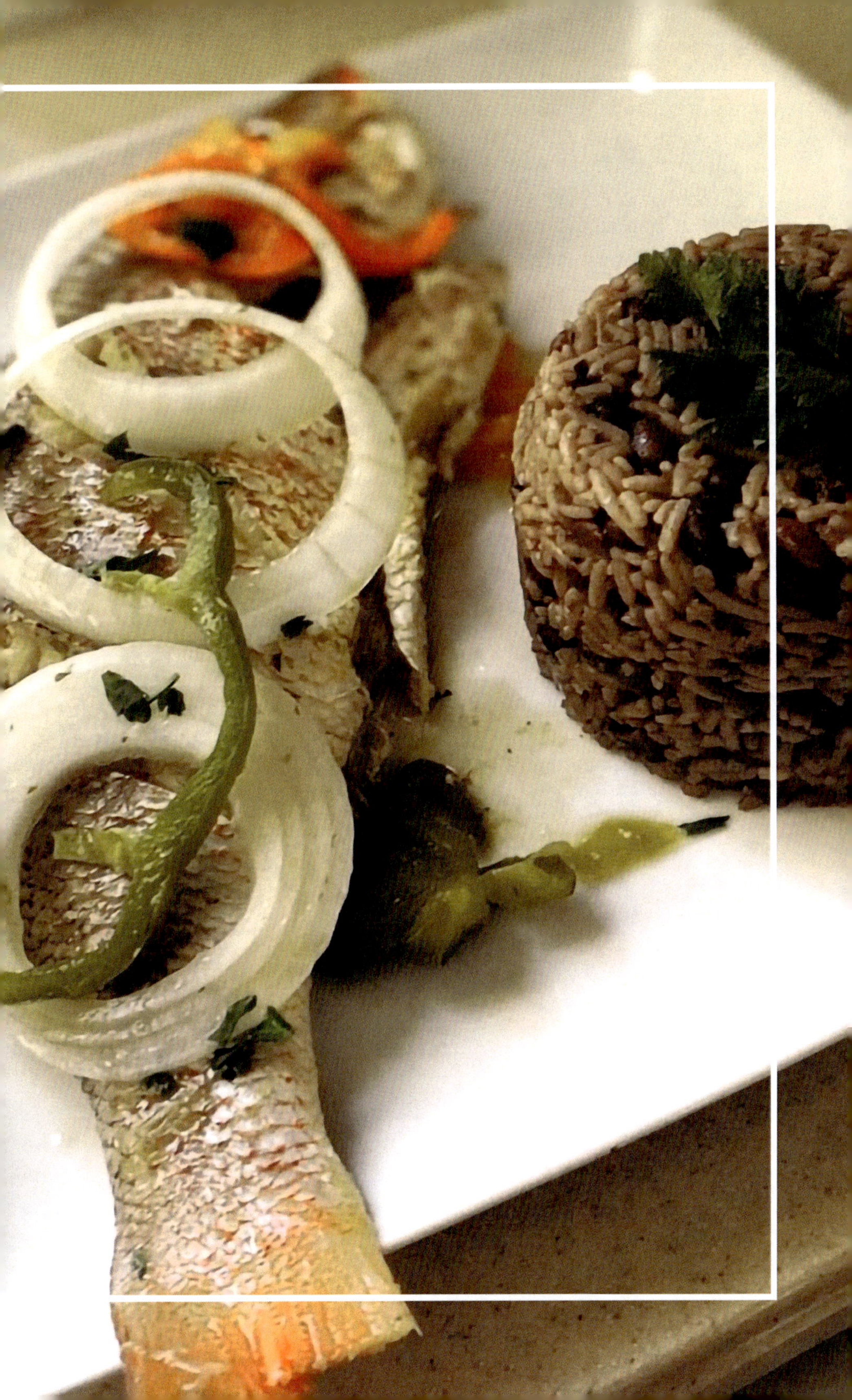

SALMON QUICHE

Quiche is the perfect type of dish for experimentation with all types of ingredients. To continue a seafood themed quiche, consider these variations: Instead of fresh or canned salmon, use smoked salmon. Use crab meat, shrimp, or lobster in place of the salmon.

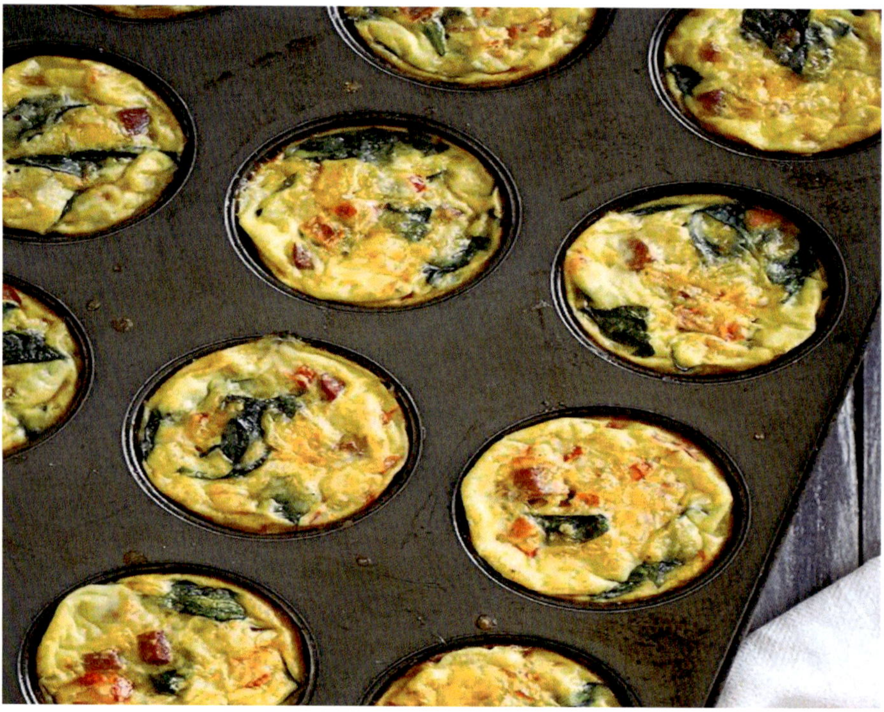

INGREDIENTS

Quiche Crust

1 homemade quiche crust

2 sheets frozen short crust pastry

1 x 9″ refrigerated pie crust, fitted in a 9″ pie dish or tart tin

1 ready-made pie shell

Quiche Filling:

15g / 1 tbsp of butter, unsalted

1 leek, white part only halved and finely sliced

2 garlic cloves, minced

8 - 10 asparagus spears

5 eggs

1 1/2 cups of cream

1/4 tsp of salt + pinch pepper

2 tbsp of fresh dill, roughly chopped

200g / 7 oz smoked salmon , cut into 4cm / 1.7″ pieces

3/4 cup of gruyere cheese

Decorations

Dill sprigs and extra smoked salmon

INSTRUCTIONS

Quiche Crust (Note 1):

1. Homemade quiche crust or frozen short crust pastry - prepare and bake the crust per Quiche Crust recipe.
2. Refrigerated pie crust - unroll, fit into a 9″ pie dish or tart tin. Bake per packet directions.
3. Prepared pie shell bake per packet directions, scale Filling down to 4 eggs

Filling:

1. Preheat the oven to 180C/350F (160C/320F fan-forced).
2.]Place cooked quiche crust on a tray.
3. Asparagus - break woody ends off. Cut into 3.5cm / 1.5″ pieces, separate tips from stems
4. Melt butter in a skillet over medium heat. Add leeks and garlic, sauté for 2 minutes, or until leeks are translucent, don't let them go golden.
5. Stir in asparagus stems (don't cook), then remove from the stove.
6. Cool slightly, then scatter across the base of quiche crust.
7. Whisk together eggs, cream, dill, salt, pepper in a bowl.
8. Scatter 2/3 of the salmon across quiche, folding/twisting pieces rather than laying flat.
9. Top with cheese, pour over egg mixture.
10. Top with remaining salmon and asparagus tips.
11. Bake for 40 minutes or until the top is lightly golden and the center is set, but still slightly jiggly when you poke it.
12. Rest for 10 minutes before carefully removing from tin and slicing.

MOFONGO MASHED PLANTAINS WITH SHRIMP

INGREDIENTS

1 15.25 Ounces of Can Whole Corn	1/2 Cup of Butter, Melted
1 15.25 Ounces of Can Creamed Corn	1 Cup of Milk
4 Tablespoons of All-Purpose Flour	1/2 Teaspoon of Salt
4 Tablespoons of Sugar	1/4 Teaspoon of cinnamon

INSTRUCTIONS

1. Preheat the oven to 350 degrees. Spray an 8X8 baking dish with cooking spray. Set aside.
2. First, make the béchamel sauce, warm the milk in a separate saucepan or in the microwave until warm to the touch, and set aside. Melt the butter in a small heavy saucepan over medium heat but not let it brown. Add the flour and stir it quickly into the butter with a wooden spoon. Cook and stir the flour-butter mixture for about 5 to 8 minutes. Pour a few tablespoons of the hot milk, just enough to moisture the flour and butter mixture. Stir thoroughly to loosen up the thick flour mixture. Add the rest of the milk to the loosened flour mixture while whisking constantly.
3. From there, you can add the cinnamon powder, sugar, salt, and cheese, to create the sauce for the corn casserole. Drain the can of whole corn and add it to the béchamel sauce and whisk together and add extra cheese on the top.
4. Bake at 350 degrees for approximately 1 hour 15 minutes or until the center is set and the top of the corn browns around the edges.

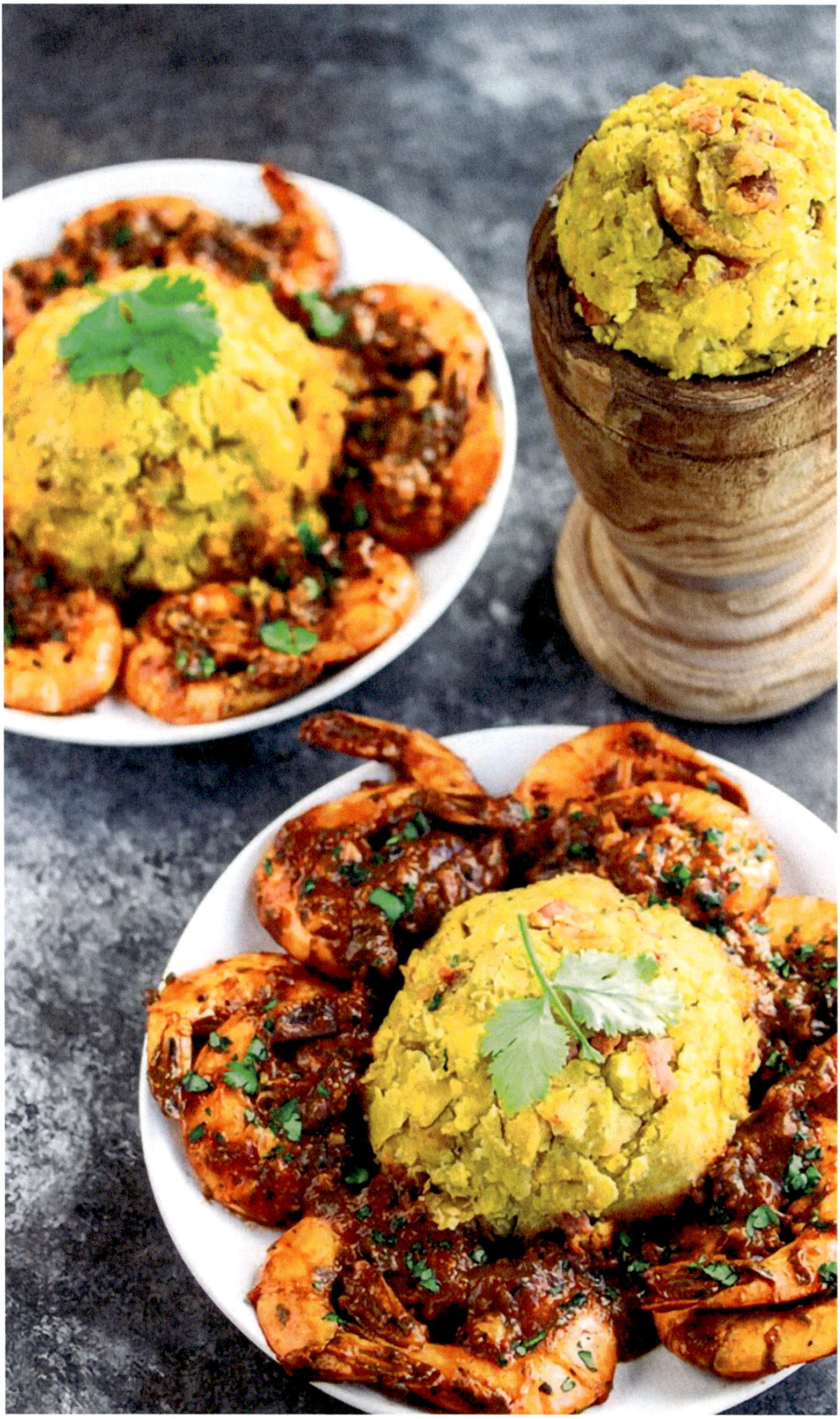

CAJUN SHRIMP & CRAB MAC AND CHEESE

This Cajun Shrimp and Crab Mac and Cheese is super creamy, cheesy, and decadent. This delicious spin of the classic dish will surely be your new favorite!

NOTES

1. *I highly recommend altering the amount of spices to YOUR taste. The amount I added was perfect for mine and my family's taste. However, that may not be the same for you, so please taste the milk and add more of the spices to your liking.*
2. *If using fresh (cooked) crab legs, remove the meat from the shell and cut it into small chunks before adding it to the pasta. You may end up with less than 2 and 1/2 cups, which is fine. The 2 pounds of shrimp make up for that!*
3. *For the evaporated milk, you can use anywhere from 2 to 2 and 2/3 cups, depending on how creamy you want the mac and cheese. I used 2 and 2/3 cups of milk because I wanted the mac and cheese to be super creamy!*

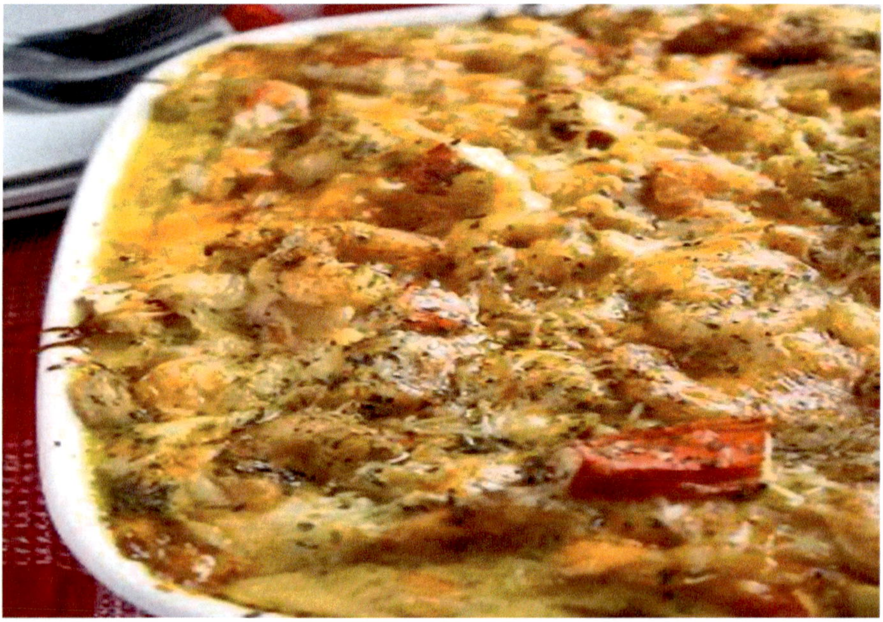

INGREDIENTS

Seafood

2 Lbs fresh crab legs

2 lbs Shrimp

Produce

1/4 cup of Basil + more, fresh or dried

Refrigerated

2 Eggs, large

Canned Goods

2 cups of Evaporated milk

Pasta & Grains

3 cups of Elbow macaroni

Baking & Spices

1/2 tsp of Black pepper, freshly ground

1 Pinch Black pepper, freshly ground

1 Cajun seasoning

1 tbsp of Cajun seasoning

1/4 tsp Cayenne pepper

1/2 tsp Paprika

1/2 tsp Salt

1 Pinch of Salt

Oil & Vinegar

2 tbsp of Olive oil

Dairy

4 cups of Cheddar cheese, sharp grated

2 cups of Cheddar cheese, mild grated

2 cups of Colby & Monterey jack cheese, grated

1/2 cup of Parmesan cheese, grated

1 cup of Whole milk

SHRIMP PIE RECIPE

INGREDIENTS

1 Pillsbury Pet-Ritz frozen deep-dish pie crust (from 12-oz package)

½ cup of chive-and-onion cream cheese spread (from 8-oz container)

4 eggs

12 oz frozen cooked deveined peeled medium shrimp, tail shells removed, coarsely chopped

½ cup of shredded pepper Jack cheese (2 oz)

INSTRUCTIONS

1. Place the cookie sheet on the oven rack. Heat oven to 375°F. Let 1 crust thaw 10 to 20 minutes. Prick bottom and around the side thoroughly with a fork. Bake on a cookie sheet 9 to 11 minutes or until very light golden brown.
2. Meanwhile, in a medium bowl, beat cream cheese spread with a whisk or electric mixer until creamy. Beat in eggs, one at a time, until mixture is smooth and well blended. Stir in shrimp and cheese. Pour into the crust.
3. Bake on a cookie sheet 30 to 35 minutes or until the center is set. Let stand 15 minutes before serving.

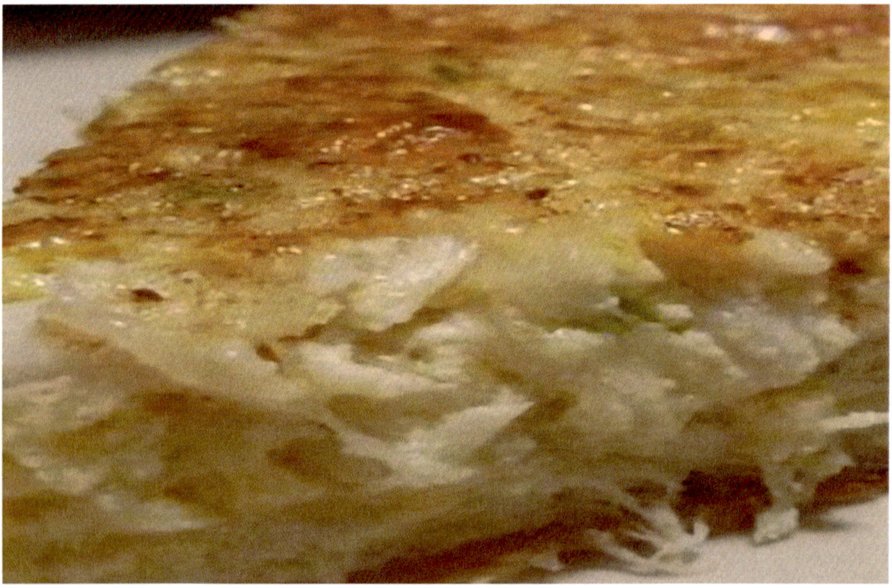

INSTRUCTIONS

For That Cajun Shrimp:

1. Browse the notes before you begin the recipe.
2. Heat a big skillet over medium heat. Inside a medium bowl, add shrimp, essential olive oil, cajun seasoning, along with a pinch of salt and pepper, and toss to mix and coat the shrimp.
3. Once the skillet is hot, add shrimp and cook, constantly stirring until shrimp is pink, 4-6 minutes. Reserve.

For That Pasta:

1. Preheat the oven to 350F (177C). Lightly butter a 9×13-inch baking dish and reserve.
2. Bring a big pot of salted water to some boil over high temperature. Add macaroni and cook until al dente (take a look at package directions to observe how long it requires). Usually, do not overcook it.
3. Drain well and transfer cooked pasta to a big bowl. Mix in Cajun shrimp, crab chunks, and basil. Reserve.

For That Cheese/Milk Mixture:

1. In a big bowl, add milk and evaporated milk and whisk to mix. Add paprika, cayenne, salt, and pepper and whisk to mix. Taste the milk and adjust the seasonings to your liking. Once your content with the taste, add the eggs and beat until the mixture is combined.
2. Reserve 1 cup of sharp cheddar cheese, 1/2 cup of Colby & Monterey, and 1/2 cup of Parmesan. Add the rest of the cheese towards the milk mixture and stir to mix.

Assembly From The Mac And Cheese:

1. Pour cheese mixture into macaroni and stir to mix. Pour mixture into the prepared baking dish. Top with reserved cheeses. Sprinkle more basil, paprika, salt, pepper, and Cajun seasoning at the top (optional).
2. Bake for 45-55 minutes or until the top is golden. Cover the very best with foil around the 35-40-minute mark, making certain it generally does not touch the cheese. Remove from the oven and allow it to sit for approximately 25-30 minutes to create before serving.

BREADFRUIT WITH OKRA

"According to an etiological Hawaiian myth, the breadfruit originated from the sacrifice of the war god ku. After deciding to live secretly among mortals as a farmer, Kū married and had children. He and his family lived happily until a famine seized their island. When he could no longer bear to watch his children suffer, Kū told his wife that he could deliver them from starvation, but to do so, he would have to leave them. Reluctantly, she agreed, and at her word, Kū descended into the ground right where he had stood until only the top of his head was visible. His family waited around the spot he had last been, day and night, watering it with their tears until suddenly, a small green shoot appeared where Kū had stood. Quickly, the shoot grew into a tall and leafy tree that was laden with heavy breadfruits that Kū's family and neighbors gratefully ate, joyfully saved from starvation."

Breadfruit made its way from Tahiti to the West Indies in the 18th century.

In Martinique, it's called: l' arbre a pain, in Saint Lucia, it's called: Bois pain and n Haiti, it is called: Lam Veritab

One single breadfruit can feed a nuclear family. The tree itself (Artocarpus altilis) produces around 200 fruits a season and grows between 85 to 90 feet tall.

"Tomtom ak Kalalau is never eaten alone. The traditional way to partake of this dish is to place the breadfruit mash in the middle of a table, the gumbo purée alongside it, and have the extended family take turns at digging into the breadfruit with index fingers, then into the gumbo sauce for flavoring, and then lightly into the mouth with one gulp until the next round. It takes a long time to eat, and this is a good occasion for conversation and stories."

INGREDIENTS

1 breadfruit

1 tsp of salt

1/4 tsp of crushed black pepper

1 lb okra (fresh or frozen)

1 tablespoon of olive oil

1/2 tablespoon of tomato paste

Chopped onions

zest of lemon

1 tsp of powdered garlic

INSTRUCTIONS

This step is very important. Peel off the green skin from the breadfruit. Cut out the most inner spongy part of the fruit. This part is bitter! Cut the fruit into pieces. Put them in a pot and let it boil for about 15 to 20 mins. It boils really fast. Make sure your pot is well covered. Make sure you have completely removed the spongy part of the fruit. Do not leave it to boil without covering it, or it might take longer to cook. You can add some salt to the boiling mixture.

1. Meanwhile, boil your okra for 10mns. Once cooked, drain water and cut into pieces. You can even mash them into a "puree." That's actually the traditional way to do it. It needs to be a slimy sauce. But I prefer mine in pieces rather than crushed (which explains the picture below).

2. Use another pot to warm your oil. Fry onions with tomato paste. Then, add your okra pieces and seasonings (garlic, salt, black pepper, lemon zest). Stir! Make sure you created a sauce. It shouldn't be dry because you want to have to dip your tomtom inside of your Kalalau. You can easily replace the powdered garlic and tomato paste with natural ingredients. The flavor will be even more amazing, and you can never go wrong with organic!

3. Now Take the pieces of boiled breadfruit and put them in a bowl that is sturdy enough. Then, use a pestle to smash them into a sticky puree.

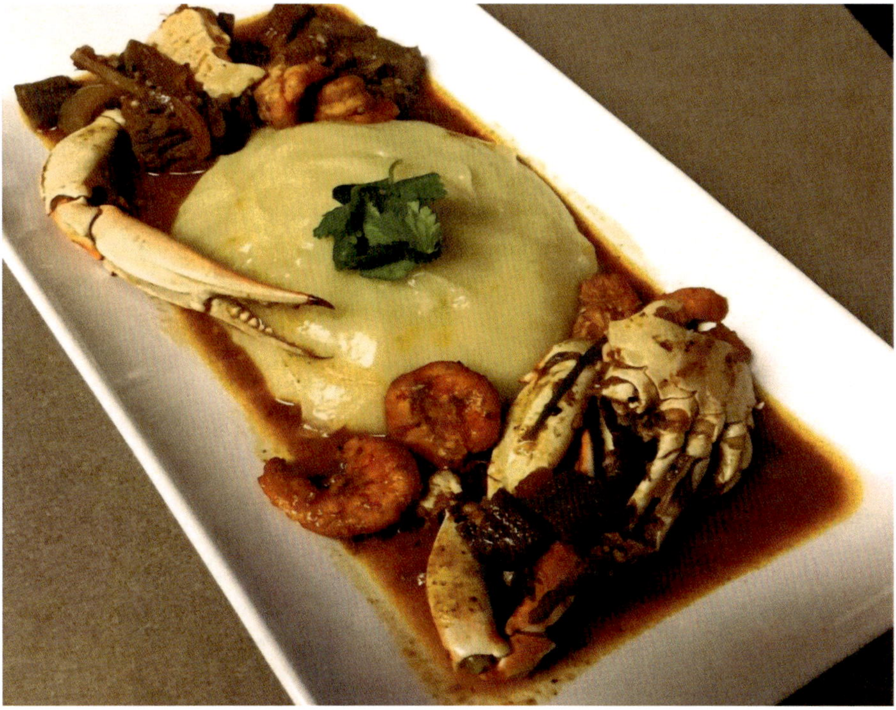

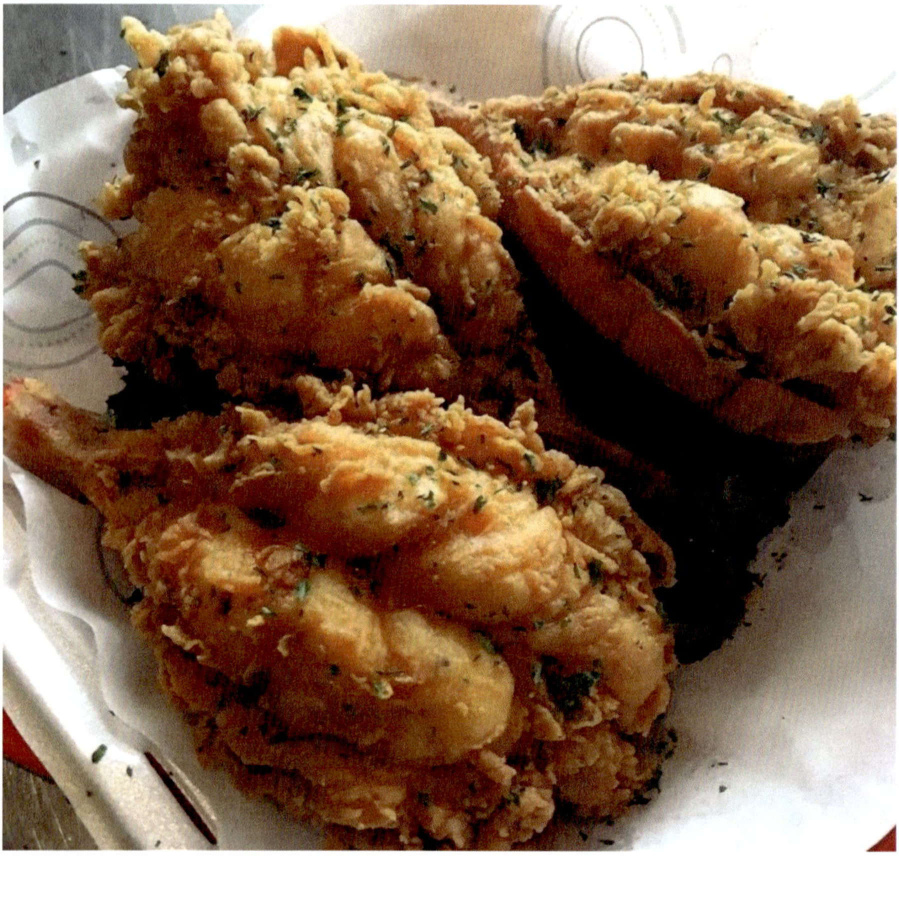

FRIED LOBSTER

INGREDIENTS

Deep-Fried Lobster

2 cups of Cornmeal

1/2 cup of Flour

Salt to taste

Pepper to taste

1 teaspoon of Cayenne Pepper

1 teaspoon of Garlic Powder

1 teaspoon of Onion Powder

4 lbs of Lobster Tails, cleaned in the shell

2 qts of Oil for deep-frying

INSTRUCTIONS

1. In a gallon-size zip-lock bag, combine the cornmeal, flour, salt, pepper, cayenne, garlic powder, and onion powder. Shake well.
2. Clean lobster tails while keeping tail in the shell. Set aside.
3. Heat vegetable oil in a deep-fryer or large, deep skillet such as a cast-iron pan. The oil needs to reach 365 degrees.
4. Place half of the lobster tails in the bag, shake well to coat the tails complete. Remove tails, set on a rack over a tray to catch any drippings and keep the work area clean. Repeat with remaining tails.
5. Deep fry one lobster tail at a time in the oil for about 4 minutes or until lightly browned. Let fried tails dry on paper towels.

RASTA PASTA WITH SHRIMP

WHAT IS RASTA PASTA

Rasta Pasta is a colorful pasta dish made with a variety of bell peppers, creamy sauce, and Caribbean seasonings, inspired by an original Italian recipe, but made with more traditional Jamaican ingredients. Because of its unique and enticing flavor, it has gained popularity worldwide, and you can find it on menus all over the world.

The name "Rasta" refers to "Rastafarianism," the powerful social movement developed in Jamaica in the 1930s. It is usually served as a vegetarian dish, as Rastafarians do not eat shellfish or meat, but many non-Rastafarian cooks add a protein to round out the meal. Jerk chicken or shrimp are the most popular, each bringing its own character to the finished dish, though oxtail is a popular addition as well.

THE ORIGIN OF RASTA PASTA

Where did Rasta Pasta come from? While many Jamaican chefs claim to have invented this classic dish, one popular story is that a chef served a mix of tomato sauce and cheese sauce thickened with coconut milk over a bed of fettuccine to a group of guests. The guests quickly drew comparisons of the textures and colors of the dish to Jamaican culture, noting the colorful bell peppers represented the colors of Rastafarianism, and the shapes of the noodles representing dreadlocks.

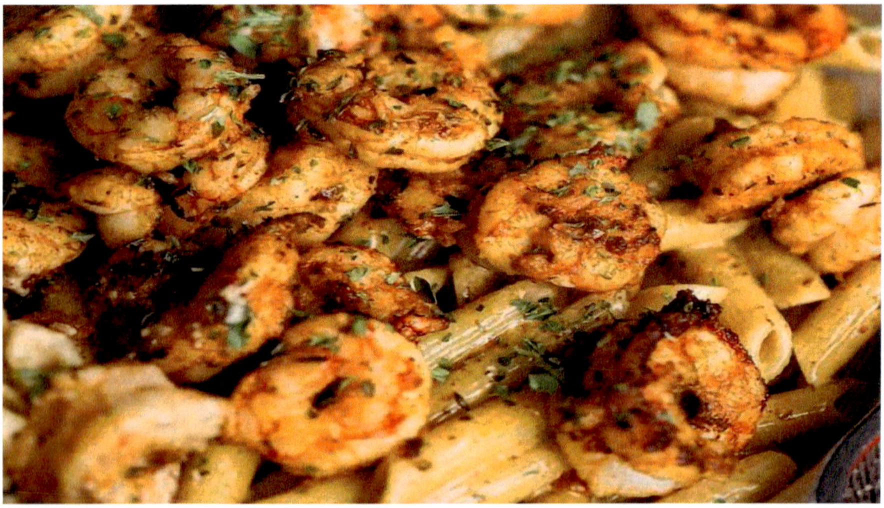

INGREDIENTS

For The Rasta Pasta

2 tablespoons of olive oil or vegetable oil

1 small onion chopped

1 green bell pepper sliced

1 red bell pepper sliced

1 orange bell pepper sliced

3 cloves of chopped garlic

1 tablespoon of Jamaican jerk seasoning

14 ounces of fire-roasted tomatoes

1 cup of coconut milk heavy cream is an acceptable alternative, yet won't bring that coconut flavor

1 cup of grated fresh Parmesan cheese or more as needed

8 ounces of fettuccine pasta

For The Shrimp

1 pound of shrimp peeled and deveined

1 tablespoon of olive oil

1 tablespoon of Jamaican jerk seasoning

For Garnish:

Fresh chopped parsley spicy chili flakes, extra grated Parmesan cheese

INSTRUCTIONS

For The Rasta Pasta

1. Heat 2 tablespoons of olive oil in a large pan and add the onion and peppers. Cook them down about 5 minutes to soften.
2. Add the garlic and 1 tablespoon of Jamaican jerk seasoning. Cook for 1 minute, stirring.
3. Add the tomatoes and stir. Cook for 5 minutes to cook down the tomatoes.
4. Add the coconut milk and simmer for 5 minutes to thicken up. If it gets too thick, swirl in a few tablespoons of water or chicken stock.
5. Stir in the Parmesan cheese and remove from heat.
6. While the Rasta Pasta is simmering, cook the fettuccine noodles according to the package directions. Drain and toss with the sauce.

For The Shrimp

7. Toss the shrimp with 1 tablespoon of olive oil and 1 tablespoon of Jamaican jerk seasoning.
8. Heat a separate pan to medium heat and cook the shrimp 2-3 minutes per side, until pink and cooked through.
9. Serve the shrimp over the pasta. Garnish with fresh chopped parsley, spicy chili flakes, and extra grated Parmesan cheese

NOTE:

Alternatively, you can tuck the shrimp into the sauce along with the tomatoes and let them simmer with the sauce until cooked through. I prefer the shrimp seared and served over the top

BLACK SEAFOOD SPAGHETTI

Haitian Spaghetti is made with spaghetti, hot dogs, tomato paste or ketchup, and spices. The recipe can be made in different ways, not a lot of ingredients, and it does not take long to make. Unlike other recipes, the tomato paste or ketchup must be cooked in oil before the pasta is added. That is how the pasta gets its color.

A lot of Haitian altered the recipe by changing the hot dogs for other types of meat links like Italian sausage, chicken sausage, cut up ham meat or turkey sausage, smoked herrings that must be de-salted before cooking, or basically no meat depending on your mood. Haitian Spaghetti is what you made it out to be with the ingredients you use. The main goal is to obtain the reddish color and the desired taste.

Typically in Haiti, this dish is served for breakfast and lunch. It can even be served for dinner because it is so versatile. It is a full meal and is also served with avocado slices. The pasta is not saucy because there is no sauce. And not dry either because of the other ingredients.

INGREDIENTS

1 Small Fennel Bulb	1 Garlic Clove
250 g (8.9 oz) Prawns	1 Tsp of Chili Flakes
1 Tbsp of Cooking Oil	1 Lemon
150 g (5.3 oz) Squid Ink Spaghetti	Salt to Taste

INSTRUCTIONS

1. Bring a large pan of salted water to a rolling boil.
2. Slice the fennel bulb as finely as you can; a mandolin is the best tool for this.
3. Slice the garlic as finely as you can.
4. Zest the lemon.
5. Add the chili flakes, half the lemon zest, the garlic, and half of the olive oil

to the prawns and season well with salt.

6. Add the pasta to boiling water and cook for 60 seconds less than the packet instructions.
7. Heat the remaining oil in a frying pan over high heat.
8. Add the sliced fennel for 3-4 minutes, tossing occasionally.
9. Add in the prawns and then Sautee for 5-6 minutes for raw uncooked and 3-4 minutes for cooked and defrosted prawns.
10. Drain the pasta reserving 2 tablespoons of the cooking liquid.
11. Toss the pasta through the prawns and add the remaining lemon zest and the juice of half of the lemon.
12. Add the cooking liquid to form a nice emulsion and serve sprinkled with fennel fronds if you have some.

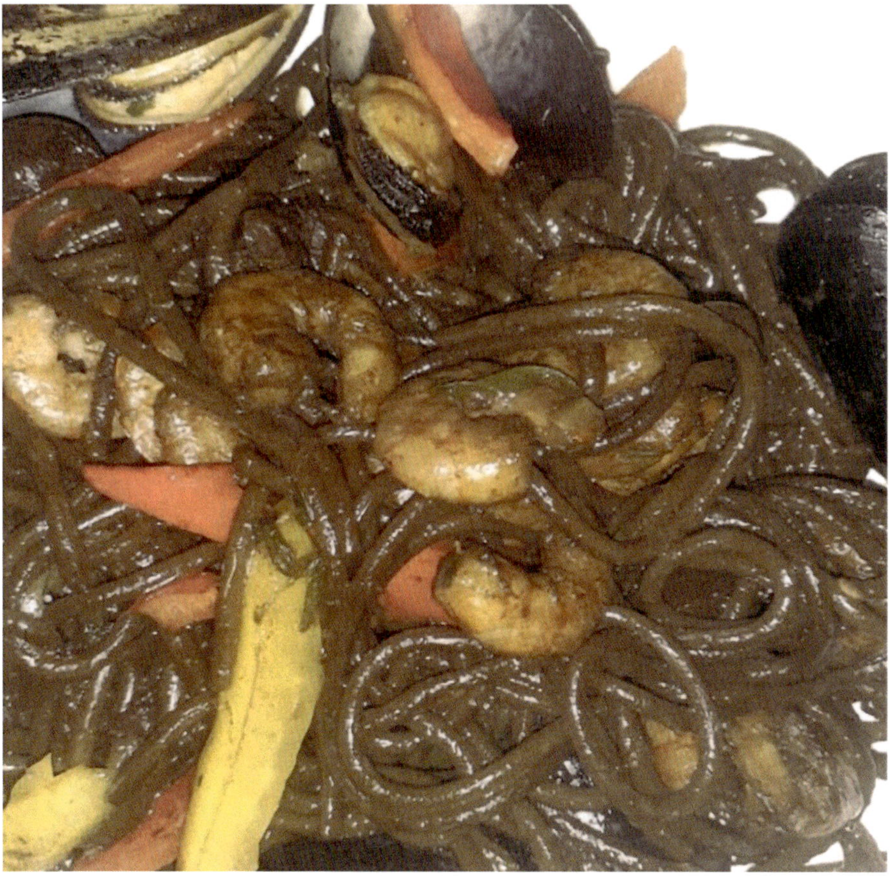

NEW ORLEANS BBQ SHRIMP

The most important thing about eating BBQ Shrimp is the sauce. You need lots of it. And lots of crusty French bread to mop it up with. Also, make note that you will get your fingers very messy and greasy peeling the shrimp. It's not pleasant, but it's unavoidable. For me, the key to good New Orleans-Style BBQ Shrimp is lots of butter, lemon juice, and Worcestershire sauce. Ironically, BBQ Shrimp has nothing to do with the barbecue. It is either cooked stove-top or in the oven. I prefer oven-baked BBQ Shrimp. The shrimp have a little longer to linger in the sauce and pick up the flavors.

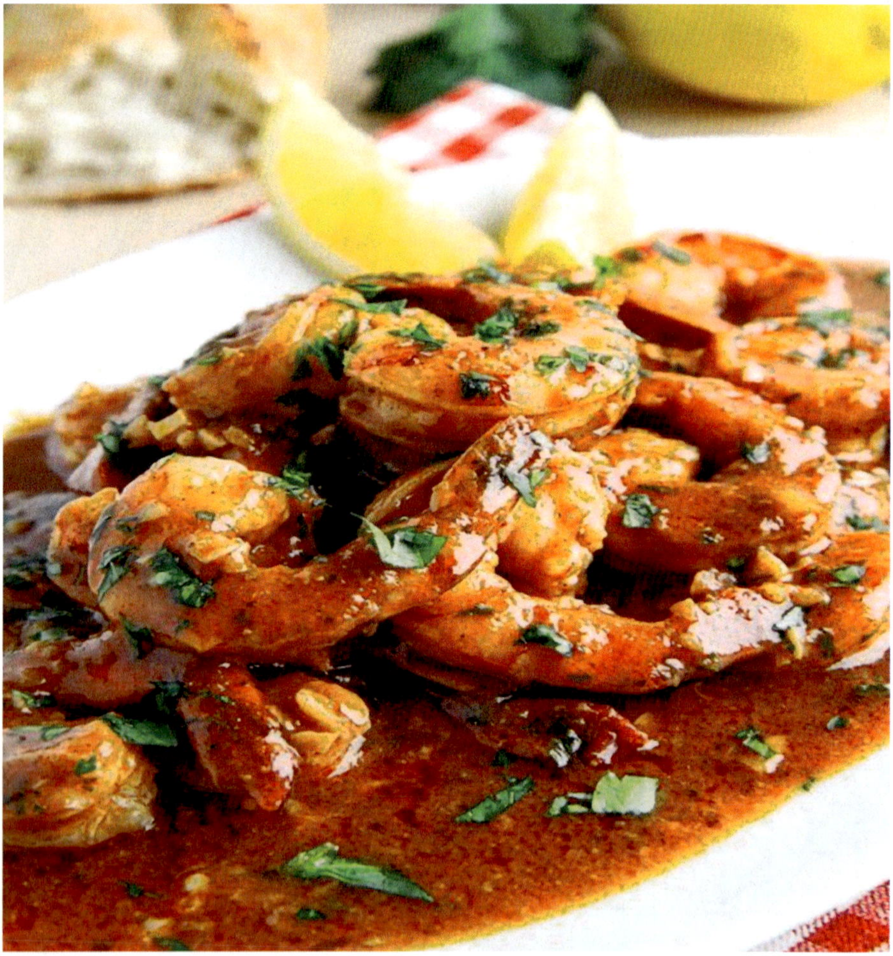

INGREDIENTS

Seafood

1 lb. Shrimp

Produce

3 cloves of Garlic

Condiments

1/4 cup of Hot sauce

2 tbsp of Lemon juice

1/4 cup of Worcestershire sauce

Baking & Spices

1/2 tsp of Black pepper, ground

2 tsp of Creole seasoning

1 Salt

Dairy

4 tbsp of Butter

Beer, Wine & Liquor

1/3 cup of Beer

INSTRUCTIONS

1. Melt the butter in a pan over medium-high heat, add the garlic, sauté until fragrant, about 30 seconds, add the hot sauce, Worcestershire sauce, beer, lemon juice, creole seasoning, and pepper, bring to a simmer and cook until the sauce is reduced by half, about 5-7 minutes.
2. Add the shrimp and cook until cooked through, about 2-3 minutes per side, depending on the size of the shrimp.
3. Reduce the heat to medium-low, stir in the chilled butter until it melts, season with salt to taste, and enjoy with French bread to soak up all of that tasty sauce!

GRILLED RED SNAPPER

Some of these red snapper recipes are easier than others. Some take longer than others to make (make sure to always check out both the preparation time and the cooking time), but they can all be done from home, completely DIY, and most of them have only a handful of ingredients that can be found at any local grocery store.

The "Veracruz-style" recipe is one of the most popular and talked about red snapper recipes out there.

It is really great because you have so many options with it, not to mention it is pretty healthy. You can make this recipe as spicy as you want by loading up the jalapeno peppers, or you can simmer it down a couple of spice levels for young kids. Either way, after you cook this easy red snapper recipe, you will quickly understand why it is so popular.

INGREDIENTS

Seafood

1 Red snapper, Whole

Produce

1/2 cup of Basil

1 tbsp of Garlic cloves

1 tsp of Ginger

1 Lemon, fresh

1 Plantain and or vegetables to grill

2 tsp of thyme

Canned Goods

1 tsp of chicken bouillon

Baking & Spices

1 tsp of Allspice, ground

1 tsp of Paprika

1 Salt

1 tsp of White pepper, ground

Oil & Vinegar

1 Cooking oil

INSTRUCTIONS

1. Make three-four diagonal cuts in each side of the fish, all the way right through the bone. Season fish with salt, pepper, and squeeze some lemon over it. Set aside
2. In a small bowl, mix all the ingredients(white pepper, allspice, minced garlic, ginger, paprika, thyme, basil, parsley, chicken bouillon, and oil) to make a marinade for fish.
3. Pour the marinade over the fish, and gently flip them back and forth until coated inside and out. Let it marinate in the fridge for up to 24hours
4. Preheat to high heat.
5. When you are ready to grill, wipe down the grill basket with an oiled towel and then immediately lay the fish down in the fish casket. Let them grill for about 1-2 minutes on each side
6. Reduce to medium-high, and then cover the grill if you have a gas grill
7. If you are using a small BBQ grill, leave the fish on the open grill or hot charcoal.
8. Baste with fish Marinate
9. Let the fish cook for a total of 3-4 minutes on each side, you may have to add a minute or two depending on the thickness of your fish until cooked – when the fish is white, and the juices must run clear.
10. Check for doneness by making sure the meat closest to the bone is fully cooked; slash with a knife to check.
11. Serve with this pepper sauce and grilled vegetables or plantains
12. Peel plantains
13. Slice in the middle then cut in halves. Season with salt and brush with a spice mix
14. Grill on each side for about 3 minutes until fully cooked through. Watch carefully because they burn easily.

CREOLE RED SNAPPER

Fish is a favorite on islands and easily found along coastal regions. The bounty of the sea is a blessing, and those who live in close proximity to the sea can find fresh and delicious choices of fish, shrimp, lobster, and shellfish around the year. If you are lucky enough to find freshly caught fish that has never been frozen, you are definitely in for a rare treat. Although this dish can be made with fish fillets, it is much better made with a whole fish, as the texture and flavor are by far superior.

In Haiti, poison gross sell is a very popular fish dish. It is a simple poached fish cooked in an aromatic broth. There are a few seasonings and spices which transform into a light citrus broth. It is traditionally served with boiled green plantains, yams, or breadfruit, although it also goes well with steamed rice. The word gross sell is the term for rock salt, which was traditionally used in this dish. Note that this fish is neither salted nor salty; it's simply the name of the dish as per tradition.

There is neither coconut milk nor tomato paste in the broth, which results in a light-colored cooking liquid or court bouillon, which is served alongside the fish. In many Caribbean islands, fish stews are cooked with tomatoes and onions in a zesty sauce. This is different and is an example of the French Creole style. Unlike traditional French court-bouillon poaching liquids, this creole version does not use white wine or juniper berries and has less liquid than the regular amounts in a poaching liquid. The outcome is light, flavorful, and tasty.

Medium size whole fish or smaller fish are probably best as you must take into consideration the size of the fish to be cooked whole. The bigger and longer the fish, the more problematic for cooking them whole; unless you own a rectangular fish poacher.

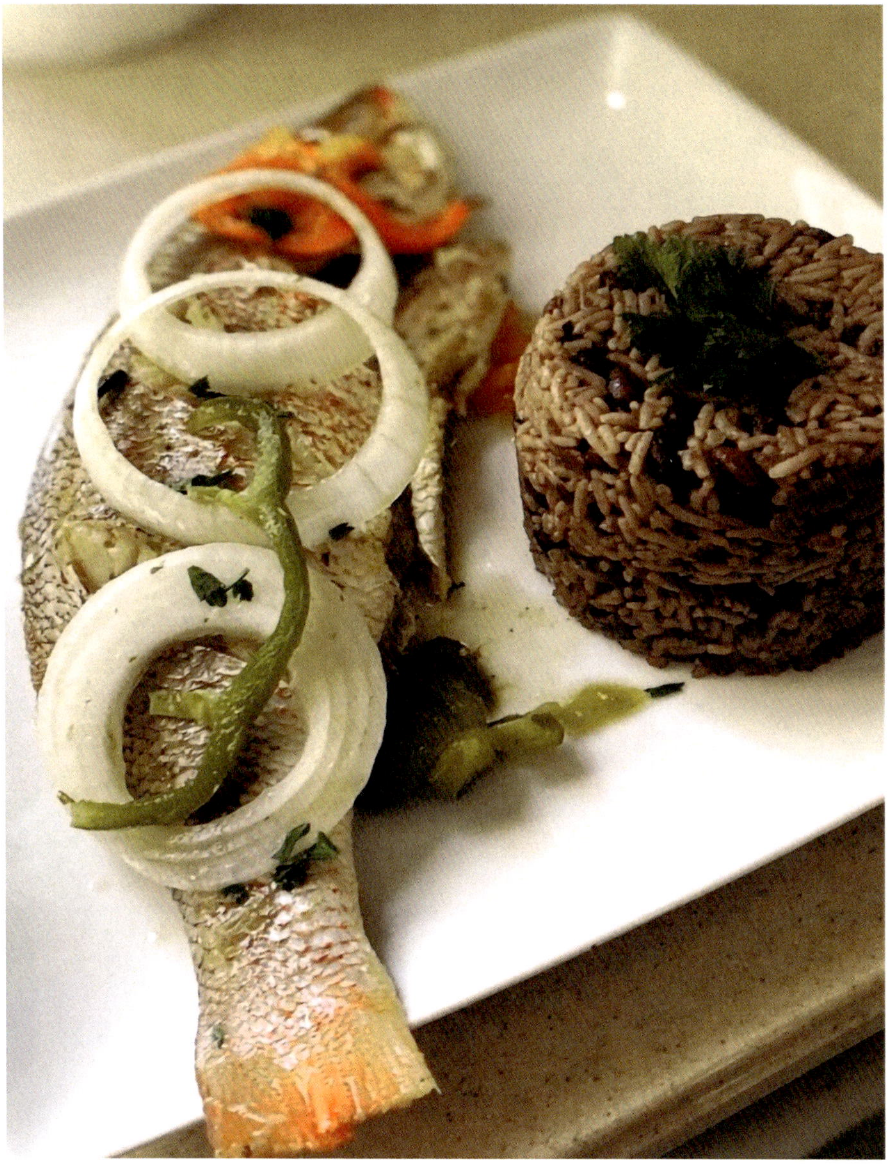

INGREDIENTS

4 small whole fish like red or grey snapper, captained, trout or parrot fish, etc. around 1lb each, cleaned, scaled, and gutted (1 per person). You can also use a large fish cut into 4 pieces.

1 cup of small Shallots or 1 medium purple onion sliced

1/2 Sweet pepper red, ½ green sliced

1 carrot julienned

3 sprigs of thyme

1 Hot pepper, whole

2 sprigs of Parsley

1 bay leaf

2 tbsp of Butter

2-3 tbsp of Green seasoning; (pureed garlic, parsley, celery, thyme, green onions or cive)

Juice of 2 Limes or approximately 1/8 cup of juice

1 tsp of Salt

½ tsp of Black pepper

2 tbsp of Olive oil

1 – 1 1/2 cups of water

1 Bouillon cube* if desired

INSTRUCTIONS

1. Season the fish with green seasoning. If using whole fish, make 2 to 3 slices on each side to allow the seasoning to penetrate and flavor the fish. Marinate for at least 30 minutes.
2. Heat a large casserole and add olive oil. Sauté the carrot slices, sweet peppers, onion, or shallots for about 3 minutes. Reserve half of the quantity to place atop the fish.
3. Place the fish onto the vegetables. Add the bouquet garni of thyme, celery, and parsley as well as the whole hot pepper.
4. Drizzle 3 tbsp of lime juice over the fish.
5. Add the butter in small cubes and 1 cup of water. If using a bouillon cube, you may crumble into the cup of water at this point and dissolve. Pour over the fish and cover with a tight lid.
6. Allow the fish to steam for about 10 minutes over medium heat.
7. Turn the fish over gently and add the reserved vegetables. Add a bit more water to ensure that there is a fair amount of sauce in the pot.
8. Add a little salt and black pepper to taste. Baste the fish with sauce. Cover the casserole and cook for 5-7 minutes additional.
9. Cooking time will vary according to the size of the fish and pieces. Generally, these smaller fish or pieces should take around 15 minutes maximum of cooking time. If using a large whole fish (3lb), it will definitely take a bit longer, around 20 minutes, give or take a few. Cook on medium heat to better control that the fish does not overcook. If slightly undercooked, the fish will continue to cook in the residual heat for a few minutes.
10. Taste sauce for salt and acidity. If needed, adjust accordingly.
11. Gently remove the fish with a large spatula and spoon the sauce and vegetables over. Do not serve the bouquet garni.
12. Perfect with boiled green plantains, sweet potatoes, breadfruit, or yams. Also delicious with steamed white rice.

NEW ORLEANS STYLE CHICKEN SHRIMP GUMBO

Just as Louisiana is a melting pot of people and cultures, this pot of gumbo combines many ingredients to make this rich and hearty stew. That's why gumbo is the official dish of Louisiana.

Gumbo is a thick stew consisting of meat, the "Holy Trinity" of vegetables (celery, onions, and bell peppers), stock, and seasonings. Every family has its own version of gumbo, and people feel strongly about what should be included. And, just like my Cajun Jambalaya, this gumbo feeds a crowd.

INGREDIENTS

Meat

2 lbs Chicken skinless chicken thigh

8 oz Sausage, smoked

Seafood

1/2 lb Crab legs

1 lb Shrimp

Produce

2 Bay leaves

1 cup of Celery

2 tsp of Garlic

1 green bell pepper, medium

2 Green onions

1 Onion, medium

1/4 cup Parsley

1 tbsp of Thyme, fresh or dried

1 14- oz can Tomatoes

Canned Goods

1 cube or 1 tablespoon of chicken bouillon powder or

6 cups of Chicken stock

1 tbsp of Gumbo file

Baking & Spices

1/2 cup of Flour

1/2 tbsp of Paprika, smoked

Oils & Vinegars

1/4 cup of Canola oil

Dairy

1/4 cup of butter, unsalted

INSTRUCTIONS

1. Assemble the cajun seasoning: Combine and mix the cajun seasoning ingredients in a small bowl. Set aside.
2. Make the roux: Heat canola oil in a large pot or dutch oven (at least 5 quarts) over medium heat. Add butter and flour. Cook until the roux turns into dark caramel color, about 15 minutes, stirring constantly.
3. Cook the vegetables: Add chopped bell peppers, onions, and carrots to the pot with the roux. Stir until well mixed with the roux. Cook until the vegetables soften and become fragrant, about 10 minutes, stirring occasionally.
4. Simmer with liquids and spices: Add crushed tomatoes (including the liquid), chicken broth, scallions, and cajun seasoning mix to the same pot. Bring to a boil and then decrease the heat to a simmer over medium heat. Cover with a lid and let simmer for 1 hour.
5. Add shrimp, chicken, and sausage: Uncover the pot. Add shrimp and sausage to the pot, mixing well. Let simmer until the shrimp is opaque and cooked, about 5 minutes. Remove from heat and serve with rice.

EGGPLANT WITH BLUE CRABS

Legumes are a traditional Haitian dish of braised vegetables and meat that is a real crowd-pleaser. It's hearty, healthy, and worth the time and effort. The meat used in this recipe is beef and turkey, but you can really use any meat, including pork, crab, ribs, conch meat, and my all-time favorite oxtail. The same goes for the veggies. The cooking time is 2 hours, and it does require a lot of attention unless you are using a Dutch oven, but this dish is a staple in every Haitian home.

INGREDIENTS

- 8 medium Blue Crabs cleaned
- 2 tablespoons of Sour Orange Juice
- 1 tablespoon of Fresh Lime or Lemon Juice
- 1 tablespoon of salt kosher or sea salt
- 1 tablespoon of Fresh Garlic minced
- 1/4 teaspoon of Noubess Hot and Spicy Original with Herbs blend
- 1 teaspoon of Fresh Ground Black Pepper
- 4 medium Eggplants skin removed and cubed into 1-inch pieces
- 4 - 6 cups of Water
- 1 tablespoon of Tomato Paste
- 2 medium Onions sliced
- 2 cups of Tomatoes diced
- 1 Bouquet Garni parsley and thyme
- 3 tablespoons of Olive Oil
- 1 cup of water reserved from boiled eggplant
- 2 medium Green Bell Peppers diced
- 2 medium Red Bell Peppers diced
- 1 large Carrot sliced or diced

INSTRUCTIONS

1. Clean the crabs. Also, remove the tips of the legs. Rinse the crabs in water and vinegar or lemon juice with water. Add to a large bowl and marinate with lime juice, sour orange juice, black pepper, salt, garlic, and hot pepper.
2. In a large pot over medium heat, bring water to a boil and add eggplant cubes. Cook until soft. Remove from water and mash with a masher or a fork. Reserve 1 - 2 cups of eggplant water.
3. In a large pan, heat oil, add tomato paste, and mix with oil. Add onions and fry for about 1 minute. Add tomatoes, and Noubess Original Hot and Spicy with Herbs blend into the onions mixture and mix well. Add peppers, carrot, and bouquet garni and cook for about 1 - 2 minutes. Add mashed eggplant and cook for 2 minutes while stirring. Add crabs, stir to mix, and cook uncovered for 20 - 25 minutes, stirring occasionally. Additional salt and pepper to taste.
4. Serve with rice or boiled root vegetables.

NOTES

Eggplant with Blue Crab can be served with rice or root vegetables such as yucca, plantains, manioc, or yams. You may add seafood seasoning if you prefer. You may also add other types of seafood, but be careful with the texture.

COCONUT CREOLE CONCH

This mouth-watering conch flesh dish is considered a delicacy in Haiti.

INGREDIENTS

1 lb. conch

2 tbsp of lemon juice

Water

1 tsp of paprika

1/2 tsp of sea salt

1 red bell pepper, julienned

1 celery heart, chopped

2 tsp of garlic, minced

2 tsp of creole seasoning

1/2 tsp of madras curry powder

3/4 cup of coconut milk

1 tbsp of olive oil

Salt to taste

INSTRUCTIONS

1. Pound conch, then cut into bite-size pieces and place in a bowl. Mix 2 tbsp of lemon juice, 1/2 tsp of salt, and 2 cups of water; pour the mixture over the conch, and let sit for 30 minutes.
2. Pressure cook with 1 tsp of garlic and paprika for 30 minutes. Turn off the pressure cooker and make sure all the steam is emitted before opening. Remove conch and set aside on a platter.
3. Sauté pepper, garlic, and celery in olive oil.
4. Stir in coconut milk, creole seasoning, and curry powder and bring to a boil. (add salt to taste)
5. Add conch to the pan and continue stirring for 5 minutes
6. Turn off heat and serve hot

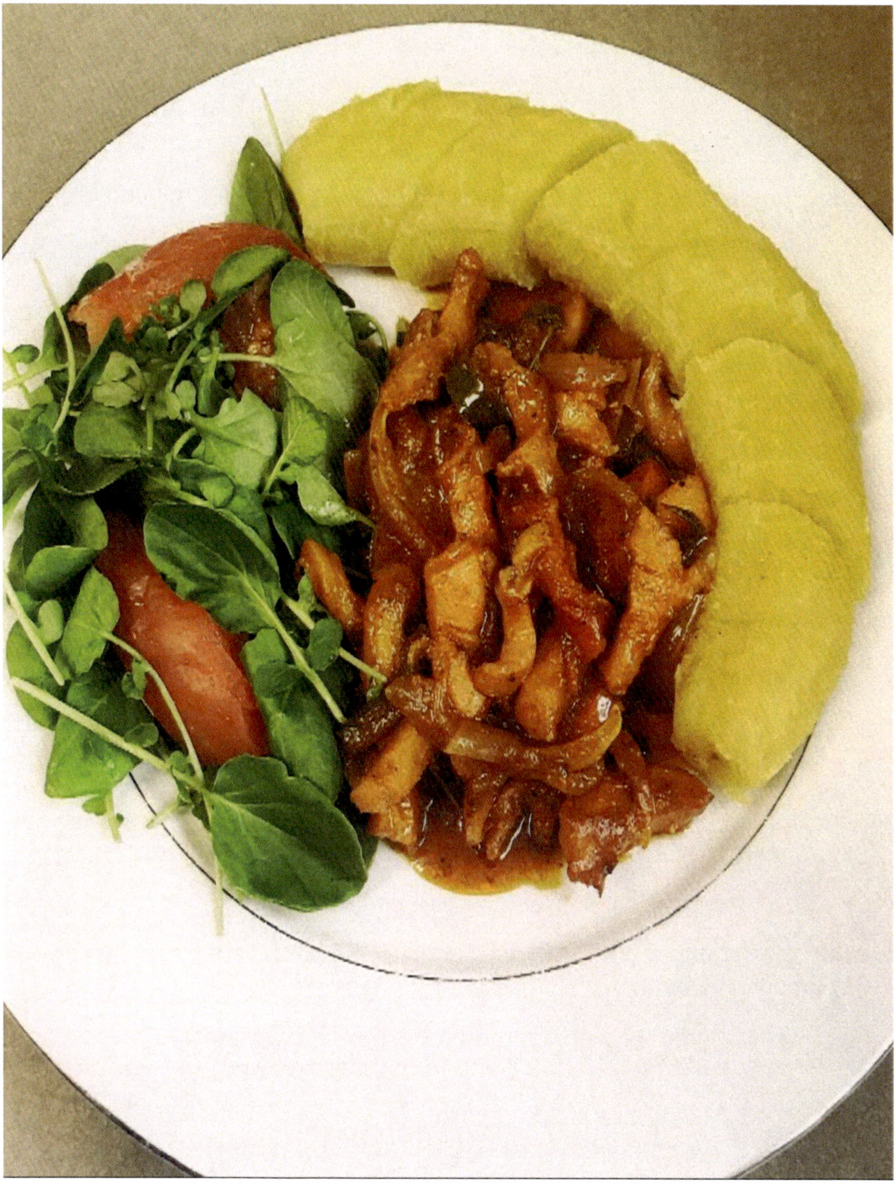

HAWAIIAN GARLIC SHRIMP

Hawaiian Garlic Shrimp have so much garlic flavor and are best served over a bed of white rice to soak up the garlic sauce. This easy appetizer or meal can be made in just minutes.

INGREDIENTS

- 1 pound of jumbo shrimp with shell on (cleaned and deveined)
- 2½ tablespoons of all-purpose flour
- 2 teaspoons of paprika
- 1½ teaspoons of sea salt
- 1 teaspoon of black pepper
- 18 large garlic cloves minced
- 2 tablespoons of extra virgin olive oil, divided
- 1 stick of unsalted butter
- Fresh chopped parsley (optional for garnish)

INSTRUCTIONS

1. Place the flour, paprika, salt, and black pepper in a large resealable bag.
2. Add the shrimp to the bag and coat the shrimp with the flour mixture. Make sure all the shrimp are coated evenly. Set the shrimp aside.
3. Melt the butter and one tablespoon of olive oil on medium heat in a large pan. Once the butter has melted, add the chopped garlic to the melted butter & oil, and cook for 2 to 3 minutes until you see the garlic has turned light brown. TAKE CARE TO NOT BURN THE GARLIC!
4. Remove the garlic sauce from the pan and set aside.
5. Add the second tablespoon of olive oil to the pan. Once heated, add your shrimp to the pan.
6. Cook the shrimp over medium-high heat for 2 to 3 minutes on each side. You may need to cook the shrimp in batches to avoid overcrowding the pan.
7. Once you have cooked the last batch of shrimp, add all the shrimp back to the pan and pour over the garlic sauce. Stir to combine and garnish with parsley.
8. Serve Hawaiian Style with sticky white rice and macaroni salad!

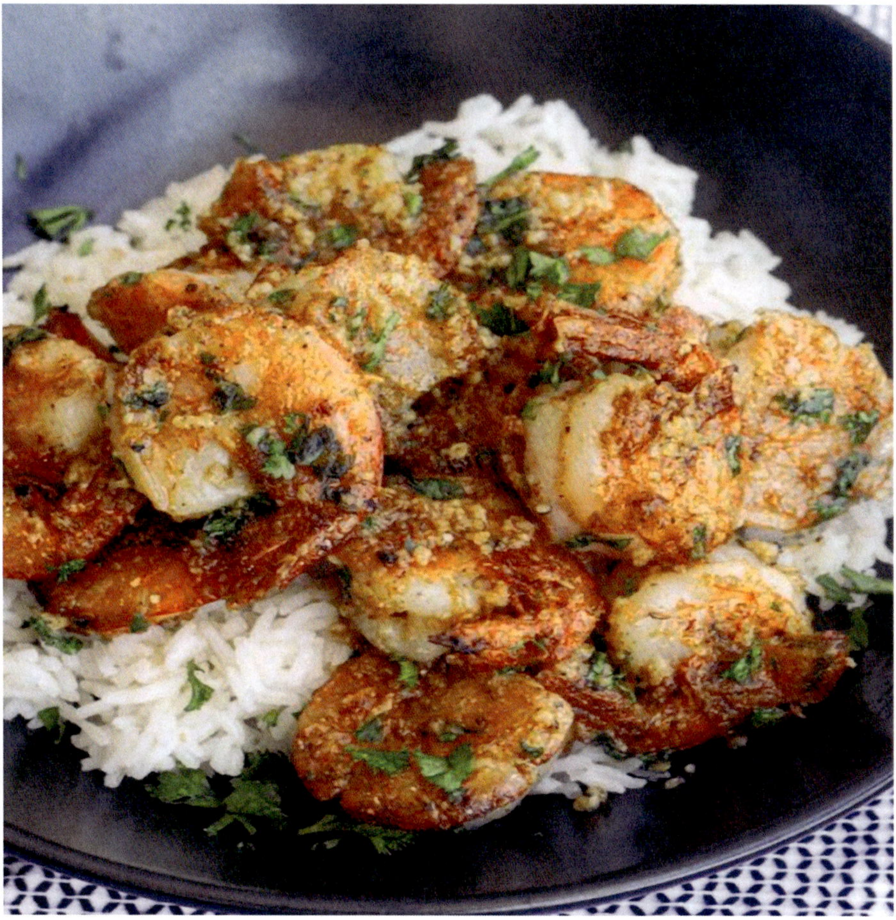

DEEP-FRIED CLAMS

Fried clams are easy and delicious to make at home with or without a deep fryer. The cracker crumb coating is seasoned with herbs and a touch of chipotle Chile pepper for a kick. Serve as an appetizer or entree.

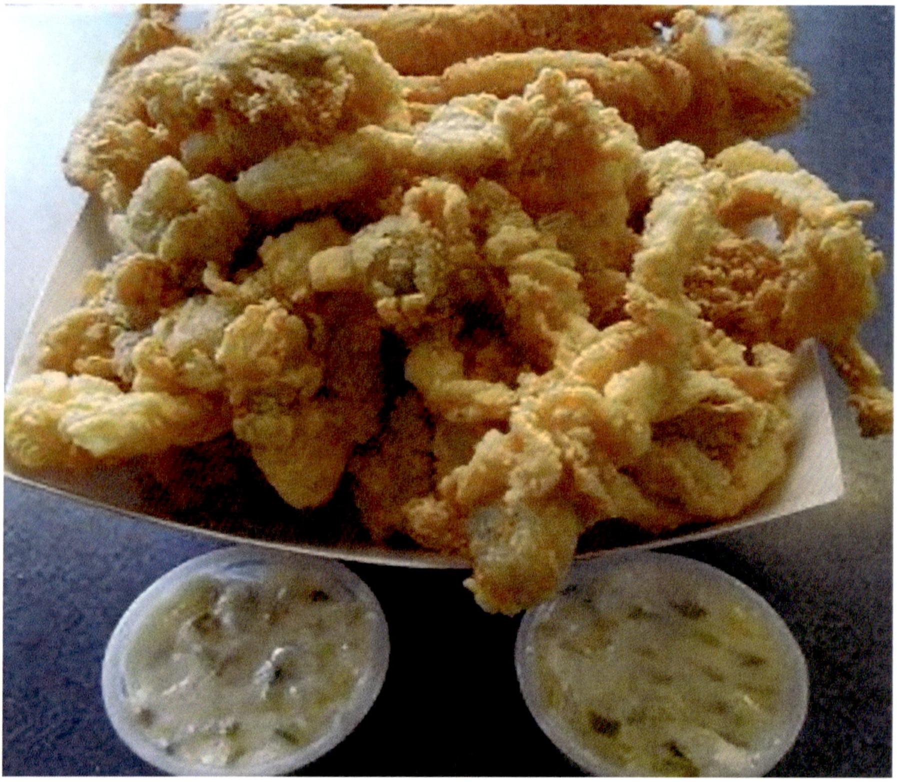

INGREDIENTS

- 2 cups of saltine crackers (finely crushed)
- 1/2 teaspoon of poultry seasoning
- 1/2 teaspoon of kosher salt
- 1/4 teaspoon of ground chipotle Chile pepper (or cayenne pepper)
- 1/4 teaspoon of garlic powder
- 1/4 teaspoon of oregano
- 1/8 teaspoon of dried dill weed
- 2 large eggs (lightly beaten)
- 1 (10-ounces) can of whole baby clams (drained, or fresh clams, shucked)
- 3 to 4 cups of peanut oil (for frying)

INSTRUCTIONS

1. You must preheat the deep fryer to 375 F or heat 3 inches of oil in a Dutch oven.
2. Measure cracker crumbs, poultry seasoning, salt, chipotle pepper, garlic powder, oregano, and dill weed into a large zip-top bag. Toss to combine. Set aside.
3. Stir the clams into the beaten eggs. Using a slotted spoon, remove a few clams at a time and place in the bag of herbed cracker crumbs. Shake to coat, remove clams, and place on a platter. Repeat until all clams are coated.
4. Fry clams in batches for about 30 seconds, until golden brown. Take care not to crowd the clams while frying. Drain on paper towels and serve hot as an appetizer or entree.

MOFONGO MASHED PLANTAINS WITH SHRIMP

Mofongo is a Puerto Rican staple dish. Relatively easy to make yet big on flavor! In a nutshell, you're just lightly pan-frying plantains and mashing them with a few simple ingredients.

It's their mashed potatoes but with much more flair! It's made with green plantains, mashed garlic, and crunchy chicharron. It's rooted in the West African dish fufu, where yams or plantains are boiled and pounded into a dough-like consistency, then rolled into balls and eaten.

It has a consistency that is neither too soft nor too hard, sitting somewhere between mashed potatoes and chunky potato salad. Once mashed, the plantains are molded into the shape of a bowl or ramekin and then stuffed with garlic and bacon in its simplest form.

Fresh herbs, onions, etc. may appear in different regional or familial versions. In this form, mashed plantains are typically aside, but when stuffed or topped with braised meats or seafood, it becomes mofongo relleno, the main entree.

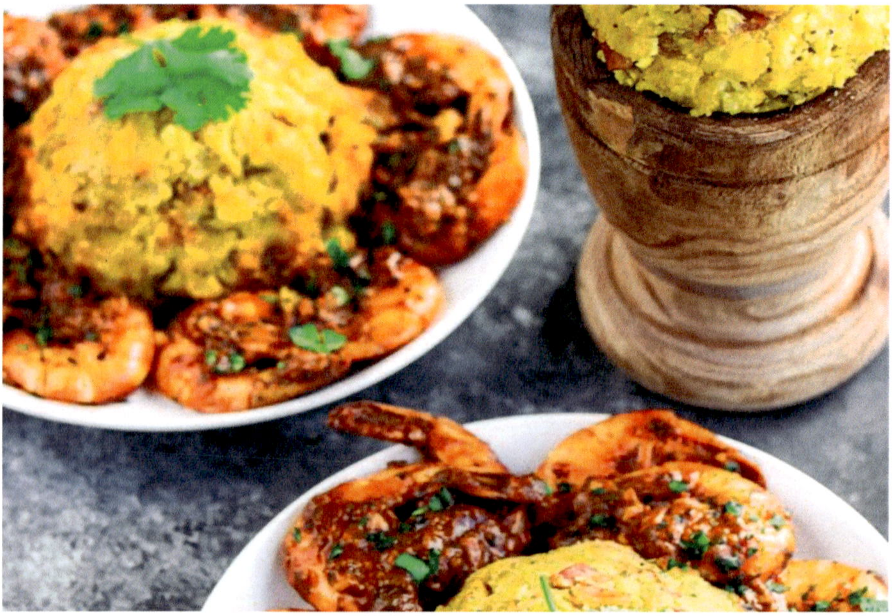

INGREDIENTS

4 whole green plantains

1 pound of medium shrimp peeled & deveined

10 pieces of chicharrónes

2 tbsp of sofrito

2 tsp of garlic minced

1/3 cup of onion chopped

8 oz tomato sauce

1/2 cup of water

vegetable oil for frying

cilantro for garnish

salt for taste

RECIPE NOTES

1. *Chicharrónes are optional or can be replaced by bacon or ham.*
2. *Minced garlic is usually mashed in the mofongo with chicharrónes, but, since the shrimp sauce is very garlicky, I prefer no additional garlic.*
3. *If shrimp sauce is too thick for preference, you may add a little bit of water.*
4. *It is best served while mofongo is still hot.*

INSTRUCTIONS

1. Begin by heating a medium frying pan of three teaspoons of oil. Add the sofrito, garlic, and onion into the pan over high heat. Sauté and stir the ingredients for three to five minutes.
2. Next, lower the heat to simmer and pour the tomato sauce into the frying pan. Also, stir in the medium shrimp and water. Set aside and stir occasionally. Once shrimp are pink, place heat to the lowest setting.
3. Heat frying oil in a separate large pan. Place piece by piece of the chicharrónes and deep fry them. Set aside over a wire rack or bowl with a paper towel to cool and soak the remaining oil.
4. Peel and chop the green plantains into 1-inch slices. Then, fry the green plantain slices until golden color. Set aside over the wire rack. Place three to five fried plantain slices inside pilón while adding chopped up chicharrónes and salt. Mash the ingredients together. You may add a little bit of the cooked shrimp liquid while mashing if the mofongo is too dry. However, make sure mofongo is dry enough to shape.
5. Finally, continue until the desired mofongo is served inside the pilón. While serving, shape mofongo into a ball and place onto the plate and flatten the top. Place shrimp over mofongo and pour the liquid over the shrimp. Garnish with cilantro and salt for taste.

SPICY VOODOO SHRIMP CREOLE

Voodoo Shrimp Creole is a spicy Cajun shrimp dish that is perfect for dinner or celebrating Mardi Gras and Fat Tuesday! Voodoo Shrimp Creole is a tomato-based dish using shrimp and beer to make a sweet and spicy broth. Serve over rice or grits for a full meal.

What is the holy trinity of creole and Cajun cooking? It is onions, bell pepper, celery, and very commonly garlic. These ingredients are sautéed together until it nearly forms a flavor-packed paste.

Voodoo Shrimp is also a spicy tomato-based dish but has the element of alcohol in the sauce. Some use beer and other Southern Comfort, a fruity whiskey. It doesn't use the trinity of creole, and in fact, it has the element of cream and a little bit of sweet from molasses-y brown sugar.

The best recipe for voodoo shrimp. This incredibly complex dish will hypnotize your taste buds. So flavorful and creamy but still low in fat. Amazing!

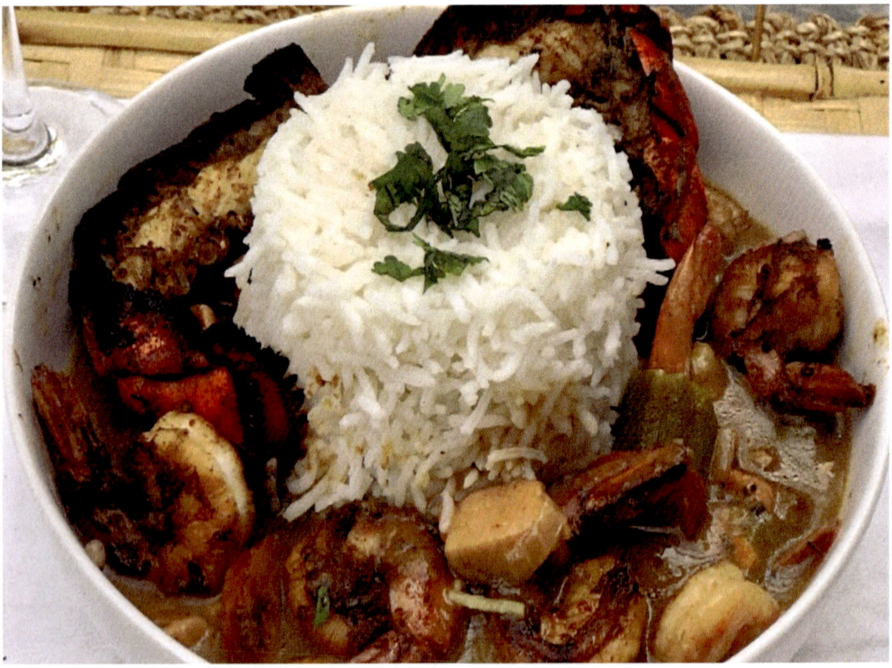

INGREDIENTS

2 tbsp of basil, fresh

3 bay leaves

2 tbsp of Garlic

2 tsp of Garlic powder

1 Lemon

½ onion, medium

1 tsp of onion powder

1 tsp of Oregano, dried

2 tsp of Parsley, fresh

1 tsp of Thyme, dried

1 (14.5-ounces) of can tomatoes, petite

Condiments

½ cup of Worcestershire sauce

Baking & Spice

2 tsp of black pepper, freshly ground

1 tbsp of brown sugar

1 tsp of cayenne pepper

2 tsp of paprika

2 tsp of salt

Olive & Vinegar

1 tbsp of Olive oil

Dairy

1 tbsp of butter

1 cup of half and half

Beer, Wine & Liquor

12 oz lager or other dark beer, black

INSTRUCTIONS

1. In a small bowl, combine paprika. Salt, garlic powder, black pepper, onion powder, cayenne, oregano, and thyme.
2. Combine 1/2 the spice mix with the peeled shrimp and mix well. Set aside.
3. Heat olive oil in a large pot over high heat. Add the onions and garlic and sauté 1 minute until fragrant. Add the shrimp shells, remaining 1/2 of spice mix, bay leaves, lemon, water, Worcestershire sauce, and beer. Bring to a boil and reduce heat to medium. Simmer for 30 minutes to reduce. Strain the liquid into a measuring cup. There should be about 1-1/2 to 2 cups.
4. Discard solids and return the strained liquid to the large pot over medium heat. Add half and half and brown sugar. Bring to a boil and reduce to 1-1/2 cups, about 10-15 minutes.
5. Add the shrimp and drained tomatoes. Return to a simmer until shrimp are pink and just cooked through, about 4-5 minutes. Stir in the butter, basil, parsley, and adjust seasoning to taste. Serve shrimp and sauce spooned over grits, polenta, mashed potatoes, rice, or toasted cornbread.

AFRICAN BAKED FISH

Whole tilapia fish seasoned the African way and grilled in the oven. Learn my special marinating and grilling technique, which ensures that the fish remains nice and moist. Serve this with some grilled plantains for the full experience. Hope you enjoy it!

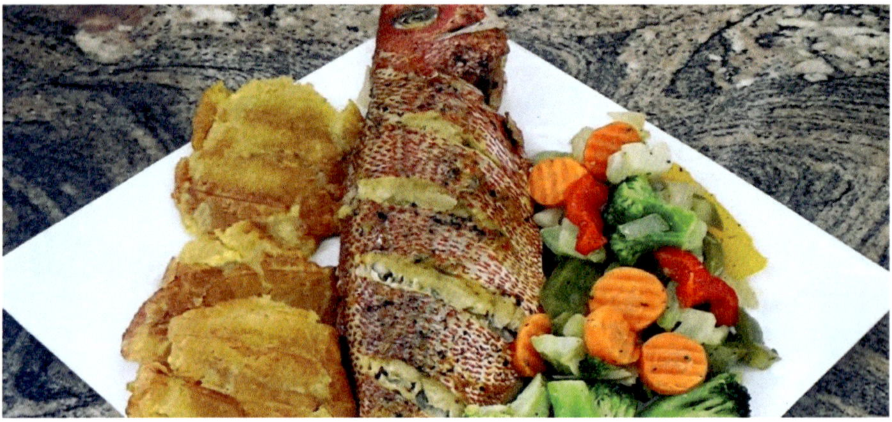

INGREDIENTS

2 whole tilapia fish - cleaned with entrails and scales removed

8 cloves of garlic - peeled

1 inch ginger root - peeled

4 stems of basil

2 stems of celery

4 stems of parsley

1 1/2 teaspoons of bouillon powder

1/2 teaspoon of salt

1/2 teaspoon of ground white pepper

2 medium onions. 1 for spice blend and 1 for garnish

1 habanero pepper (optional)

1/4 cup of oil I used peanut oil

SOME TIPS FOR MAKING PERFECT OVEN GRILLED TILAPIA

- *Use fresh herbs and spices for best flavor but if you are short on time, use dry spices and herbs mixed with oil.*
- *If you are using a gas oven, rotate your tray while broiling because gas ovens heat unevenly and will cause some portions of the fish to burn while other parts don't gain any color.*
- *For a great tasting fish, marinate the fish and keep covered in the fridge to absorb all the flavors overnight. You can then take it out and proceed with grilling the next day.*

INSTRUCTIONS

1. Combine the celery, parsley, and basil together with the garlic, ginger, and 1 onion (roughly chopped) in a blender. Add a quarter cup of water and blend into a paste. We'll call this the green spice mixture. Set the green spice mixture aside.
2. Use kitchen shears to trim the fins of the fish. Totally cut out the fins towards the tail of the fish. Also, use a paring knife to cut out the gills from the head of the fish.
3. Rinse fish thoroughly and pat dry with a paper towel. Make four diagonal cuts on each side of the fish. Sprinkle on 1/4 teaspoon of salt and 1/4 teaspoon of withe pepper. Rub well all over the fish.
4. Mix together 4 tablespoons of the green spice mixture with 2 tablespoons of oil and 1 teaspoon of bouillon powder. Rub the mixture all over the fish, being careful to fit some into the diagonal cuts.
5. Brush a baking tray generously with oil then place the fish on top. Cover with aluminum foil and let it marinate for at least 30 minutes or overnight.
6. Place fish while covered with foil to cook in a preheated oven at 400 degrees Fahrenheit (200 degrees Celsius) for 20 minutes.
7. Remove fish and take out the foil covering. Brush with a little oil, then set the oven to broil and place fish back in. This helps give the fish some color on the outside.
8. Remove fish and let it rest, then you can serve with some green sauce and your favorite side. Mine is ripe plantains!

Green Sauce for Fish recipe

1. In a saucepan, combine the remaining green spice mixture with the remaining oil and bouillon powder. Add in 1/4 teaspoon of white pepper and 1/4 teaspoon of salt. Stir to combine and cook on medium heat for about 5 minutes.

Recipe Notes

1. *Be careful not to overcook the green sauce, so it doesn't turn brown. About 5 minutes is a cook time for everything to simmer together.*
2. *This grilled tilapia is on the hot side, which means the heat from the pepper is very present. If you can't tolerate heat, omit the habanero.*

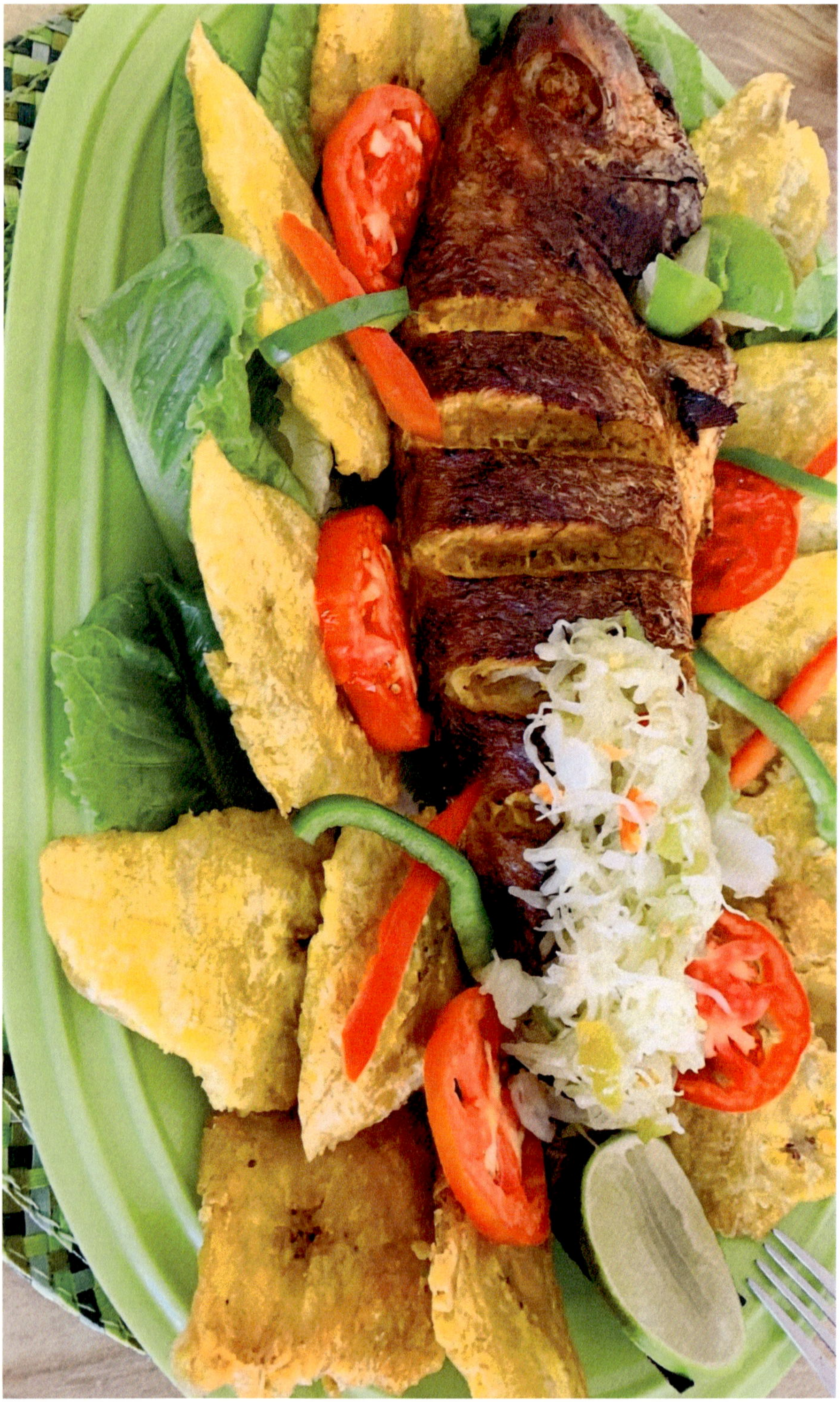

AFRICAN FRIED FISH

INGREDIENTS

Oil - for frying

First Marination:

Lemon Juice - 1/2

Salt - as required for each fish

To be ground to a fine paste and used for Second Marination:

Turmeric Powder - 1/2 tsp

Red Chili Powder - 1 tbsp

Pepper - 1/2 tsp

Ginger Garlic Paste - 1/2 tbsp

Fennel Seeds - 1 tsp

Coriander Powder - 1 tsp

Corn Flour - 1 tsp

Food Color (Red) - pinch (Optional)

INSTRUCTIONS

1. Clean and prepare the fish and marination paste. For the first marination, make small slits using a knife on both sides. Rub with salt and lemon juice on each piece. Let it sit for 10 minutes.
2. 2. Prepare the second marination paste with little water to form a fine paste. Rub the marination deep and fully over the fishes and let it marinate for 2 hours. Heat oil for deep frying, add the fishes one by one.

Notes:

The marination has to be as dry as possible, so it sticks completely to the fish.

Be careful while frying the fish.

Deep fry or shallow fry and serve hot!!!

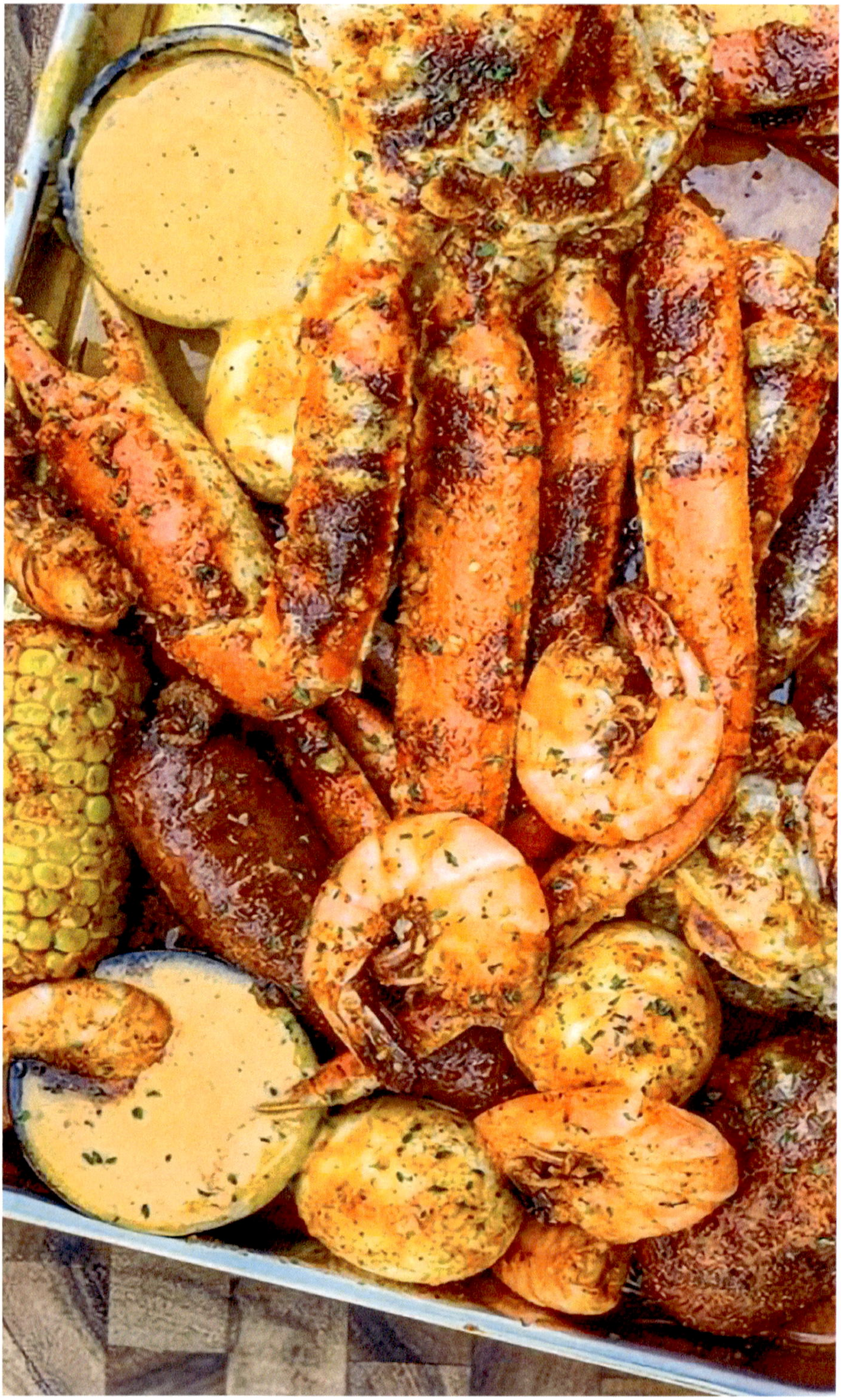

GARLIC BUTTER SEAFOOD BOIL SAUCE

INGREDIENTS

Meat

1 lb Andouille sausage, sliced thick

Seafood

5 Clusters snow crab legs

1 lb Shrimp

Produce

6 Baby red potatoes

3 Bay leaves

6 Corn, on the cob

3 tbsp of Garlic

1 Lemon, whole

1 Lemon

1 Onion, whole

Baking & Spices

1 tbsp of Cayenne pepper

8 tbsp of Old bay seasoning

3 tbsp of Paprika

1 tbsp of Red pepper flakes

Oils & Vinegars

1/4 cup of Olive oil

Dairy

4 sticks Butter

INSTRUCTIONS

1. Add all ingredients except shrimp and corn in a pot
2. Simmer until all ingredients are mixed in, tasting to your liking
3. Add shrimp, stirring continually to ensure shrimp cooks thoroughly. Don't overcook shrimp
4. Once shrimp turns pinkish, add corn and cook for 2 minutes
5. Turn off fire and cover for 5 minutes.

HAITIAN RUM & ASIAGO SHRIMP PASTA

INGREDIENTS

1 pound of whole-grain angel hair pasta, cooked & drained

3 tablespoons of olive oil

2 tablespoons of unsalted butter

1 tablespoon of salt

1/2 tablespoon of pepper

1/2 tablespoon of red pepper flakes

About 6 large garlic cloves, sliced

1/2 tablespoon of dried parsley

1/4 tablespoon of dried oregano

1/4 tablespoon of dried thyme

1/2 cup of good Haitian rum

1 1/2 cups of shredded Asiago cheese

1 pound of jumbo shrimp, peeled and deveined, but with the tails on

fresh cilantro, to garnish

INSTRUCTIONS

1. In a large skillet, heat the olive oil. When the olive oil is warm, add in the garlic and butter.
2. Once the garlic is fragrant and just lightly toasted, add in the salt, pepper, red pepper flakes, dried parsley, dried oregano, and dried thyme. Cook on medium heat for about 2-3 minutes, so the flavors have a chance to marry.
3. Then, add in the rum. To do this, remove the skillet from the flame first. Pour the rum into a cup and then add the rum to the pan. Never pour directly from the bottle, especially over the heat.
4. Once the rum has reduced by half, add in the shrimp and let the shrimp cook through in the sauce.
5. To finish the dish, toss in the whole grain pasta and Asiago cheese. Garnish with fresh cilantro.

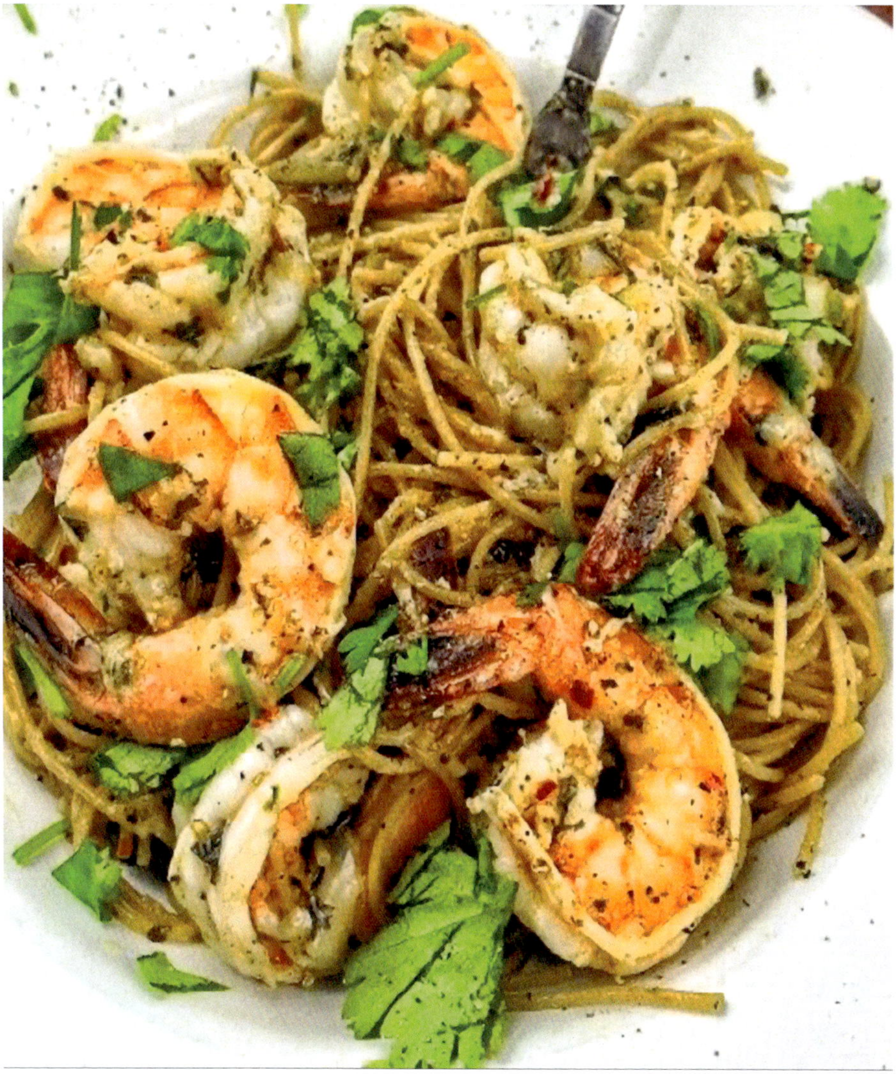

SALMON RASTA PASTA

- Use a whisk to mix the Parmesan cheese into the sauce
- Make sure you're using a good quality Parmesan cheese
- If cheese clumping, lower heat and whisk harder and allow the sauce to cook a little longer

INGREDIENTS

4 salmon filets (4-6 ounces each)

3 tablespoon of olive oil

1 medium red bell pepper

1 medium green bell pepper

3 sprigs of green onion (scallion)

3 garlic cloves, minced

2 cup of heavy cream

1/2 cup of coconut milk

1/2 cup of chicken broth

5-8 ounces of shredded Parmesan cheese

16 ounces box of rigatoni noodles

Pink Himalayan Salt

Ground Black pepper

Jamaican Jerk seasoning (Mild)

Thyme

Paprika

Parsley to garnish (optional)

Grated Parmesan to garnish (optional)

INSTRUCTIONS

Salmon

1. Generously sprinkle both sides of the salmon filets with salt, pepper, jerk seasoning, and thyme and set aside
2. Add 2 tablespoon of oil to a skillet and warm over medium-high heat
3. Add salmon, and cook on each side for about 3-5 minutes, depending on the thickness of the filet
4. Remove from heat and set aside until ready to assemble pasta plate

Pasta

1. Cook noodles according to packaging, then drain and set aside
2. In a large pot, add 1 tablespoon of oil and garlic, then cook for 1-2 minutes on medium-high heat
3. Add the red pepper, green pepper, and green onion then sauté for 5-7 minutes or until tender
4. Stir in heavy cream, coconut milk, and chicken broth and allow it to simmer for 10 minutes while stirring every few minutes
5. Generously season sauce mixture with salt, pepper, jerk seasoning, paprika, and thyme -stir well
6. Stir in Parmesan cheese and allow the sauce to cook for 5-7 minutes (taste to make sure it's seasoned to your liking-adjust if necessary)
7. Add the noodles to the sauce mixture and cook for another 7-10 minutes, stirring every few minutes
8. Remove from heat and serve!
9. Garnish pasta with parsley and grated Parmesan (optional)

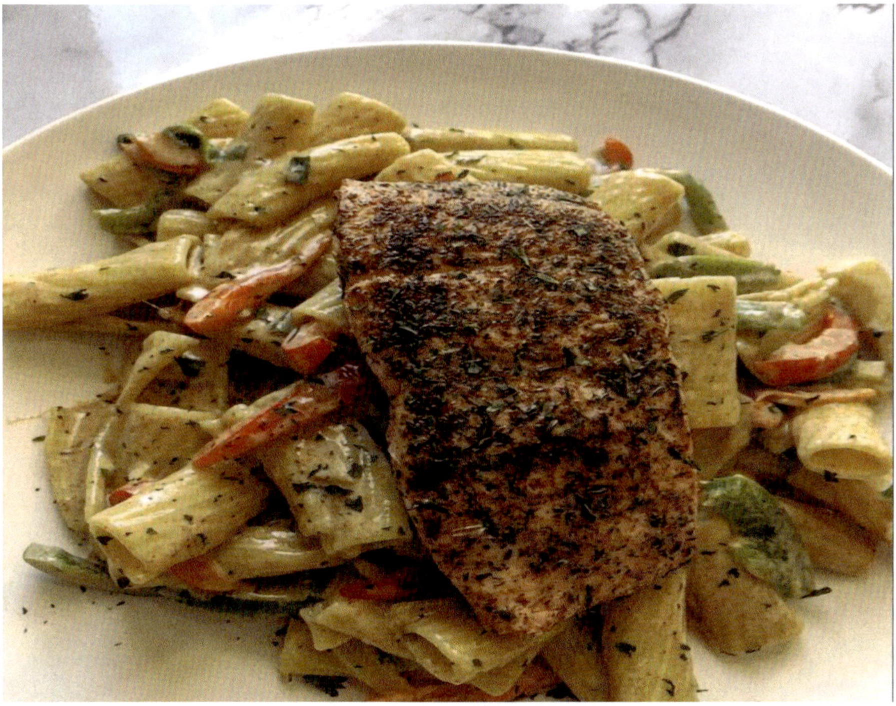

06 WEEKNIGHT DINNER

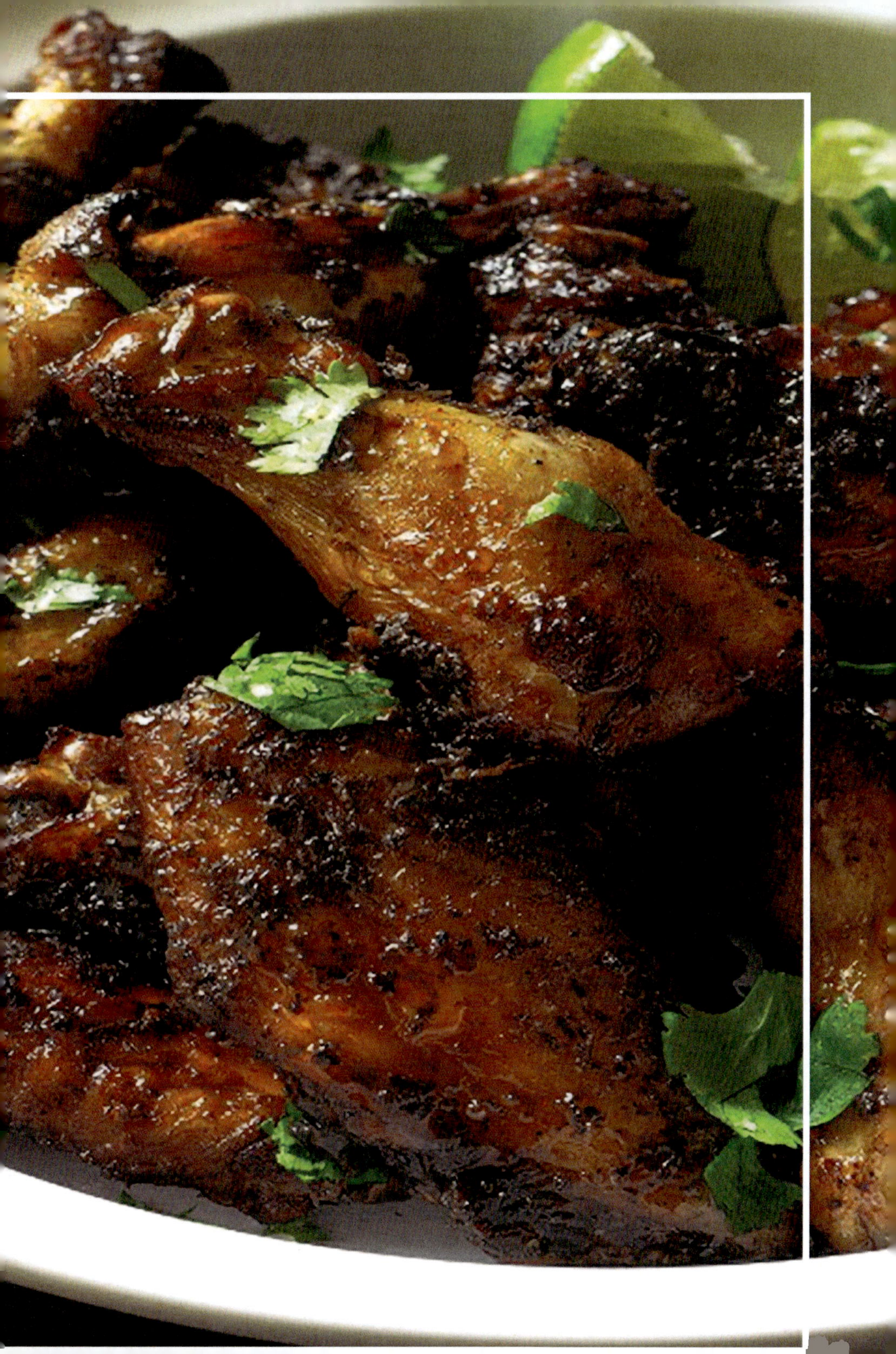

PHILLY CHEESESTEAKS SANDWICHES

No matter what variety you choose, you'll want to simply embrace the mess it creates, and here's why: After the cheese is melted and the steak is sizzling and caramelized in the skillet, you'll use a spatula to transfer the filling into the sliced rolls. It's nearly impossible to maintain the neat layers of cheese, peppers, onions, and steak and move the mound in one clean scoop. Instead, allow the filling to mix with the melted cheese as you stuff it into the bread, which, honestly, makes it all the more delicious.

INGREDIENTS

- 1 1/2 pounds of ribeye or sirloin steak
- 2 (12-inch) soft sub or hoagie rolls
- 1 teaspoon of kosher salt, divided
- 1/2 teaspoon of freshly ground black pepper, divided
- 2 tablespoons of vegetable oil, divided
- 1 large yellow onion, thinly sliced
- 1 medium red bell pepper, thinly sliced
- 1 medium green bell pepper, thinly sliced
- 4 slices of American cheese, preferably white
- 4 slices of provolone cheese

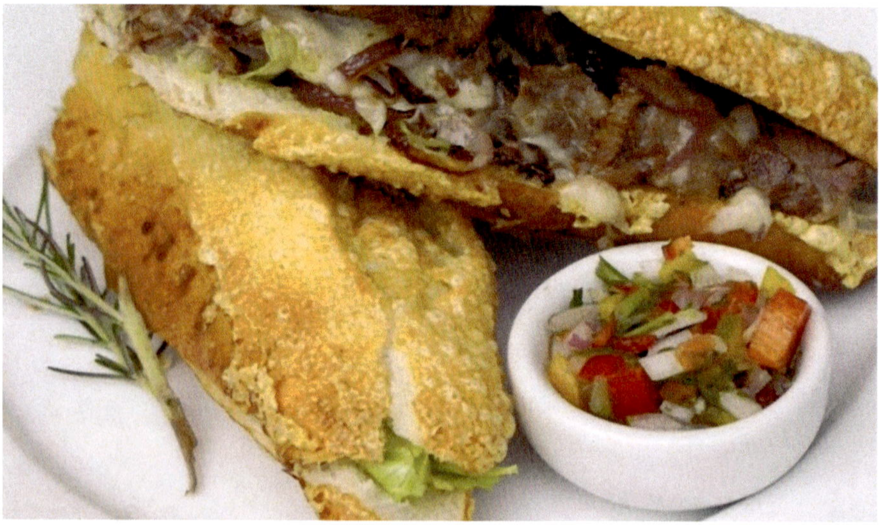

INSTRUCTIONS

1. Freeze the steak until firm. Place the steak in the freezer until very firm but not frozen, 2 to 3 hours.
2. Slice the rolls. Slice the rolls lengthwise, leaving one side attached. Set aside.
3. Slice the steak into 1/8-inch thick strips and season with salt and pepper. Remove the steak from the freezer and slice crosswise into very thin (1/8-inch thick) strips. Season the steak with 1/2 teaspoon of the salt and 1/4 teaspoon of the pepper; set aside.
4. Sauté the onion and bell peppers. Heat 1 tablespoon of oil in a large skillet over medium-high heat until shimmering. Add the onion, bell peppers, remaining 1/2 teaspoon of salt, and 1/4 teaspoon of pepper and cook until the onions are soft and browned, and the bell peppers are tender 15 minutes. Transfer the vegetables to a plate, cover with aluminum foil, and set aside.
5. Cook the steak until browned. Heat the remaining 1 tablespoon of oil in the skillet over medium-high heat until shimmering. Add the steak and cook for 1 minute without stirring. Stir and repeat until all the steaks are browned, 7 to 9 minutes total cook time. After browning the meat, some moisture will remain in the pan.
6. 6. Top the steak with vegetables and cheese. Divide the steak into two piles and top each pile with the onion and pepper mixture. Arrange the cheese slices over the top, alternating the American and provolone cheeses.
7. Cook until the cheese melts, and the steak is crispy. Cook until the cheese melts and the bottom layer of steak is browned and crispy, about 6 minutes.
8. Scoop the filling into rolls, then slice the sandwiches in half. Use a thin, flat spatula to scoop one pile of cheesesteak filling into each roll. It is ok if it takes a few scoops to transfer the filling because as you scoop, the steak, vegetables, and cheese mix together. There is no need to maintain the layers or transfer in a single scoop at this point. Use a serrated knife to slice each roll in half.

SLOW COOKER JAMAICAN JERK CHICKEN CHILI

INGREDIENTS

For The Jamaican Jerk Chicken Chili:

2 – 2 1/2 pounds of boneless, skinless chicken breasts or thighs

8 sprigs of green onion, plus more, to top

1 large white onion, diced

3 bell peppers, diced (I like to use one red, one green, and one yellow)

1 habanero pepper, finely minced

1 (15 ounces) can kidney beans

1 (15 ounces) can black beans

1 (28 ounces) can crushed tomatoes

6 cloves of garlic, minced

1 cup of mild Jamaican jerk marinade

1/4 cup of low sodium soy sauce

1 tablespoon of brown sugar

2 teaspoons of kosher salt

2 teaspoons of dried thyme

2 teaspoons of cumin

2 teaspoons of ground allspice

1 teaspoon of black pepper

1/2 teaspoon of cinnamon

Juice of 3 limes

1/4 cup of chopped cilantro

Shredded cheddar cheese, to top

Sliced avocado, to top

For The Plantain Chips:

3 larges unripe (green) plantains

Vegetable oil, for frying

Coarse sea salt

INSTRUCTIONS

1. Combine the chicken, onions, peppers, beans, crushed tomato, garlic, Jamaican jerk marinade, soy sauce, salt, brown sugar, thyme, cumin, allspice, black pepper, and cinnamon in a large slow cooker. Stir gently to ensure that the spices are distributed.
2. Cover the slow cooker and cook on low for 6-8 hours, or on high for 4 hours. In the meantime, make the plantain chips. Cut off the ends of the plantains and cut shallow, vertical slits on each side of the skin of each plantain. Microwave for 1 minute at 50 percent power. Pull off the peel of each plantain, and then slice into 1/8" thick slices using a mandoline.
3. In a large, heavy-bottomed pot, heat an inch and a half of oil to 350°F over medium heat. Working in batches, carefully add the plantain slices to the hot oil. Cook until golden brown, occasionally turning for about 4-5 minutes. Using a slotted spoon, transfer the plantain chips to a paper towel-lined plate to drain and cool. Then, sprinkle with sea salt. Set aside until ready to serve.
4. When the chili has cooked, remove the lid, stir, and shred the chicken. Then, mix in the lime juice and cilantro. Taste and adjust seasonings accordingly.
5. Serve warm with additional green onion, shredded cheese, and sliced avocado, if desired.

NOTES

If you'd like your chili to be very spicy, feel free to add in an extra habanero pepper. Keep in mind that the spiciness of your Jamaican jerk marinade will affect the heat level of your chili, and adjust accordingly if necessary. My marinade was relatively mild.

FRIED CHICKEN CORNBREAD CAKE

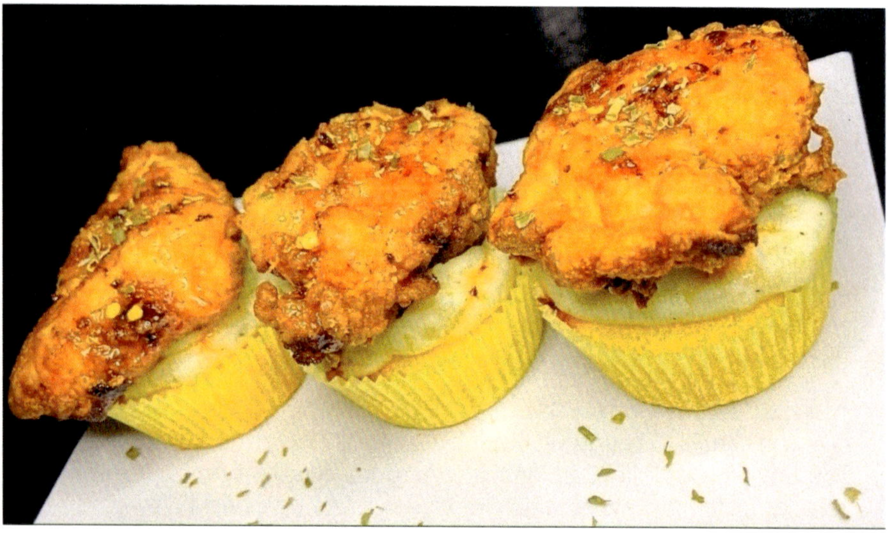

INGREDIENTS

Cornbread Recipe

cup of all-purpose flour

1/2 teaspoon of baking soda

1 cup of cornmeal

1/2 cup of granulated sugar

1/2 teaspoon of salt

1/2 cup of butter (melted)

2 eggs

1 cup of buttermilk (if you don't have buttermilk, mix 1 tablespoon of lemon juice or 1 tablespoon of vinegar with 1 cup milk)

Garlic & Thyme Mashed Potato Recipe

3 large Russet potatoes (peeled, quartered, and boiled until fork tender)

1 tablespoon of olive oil

2 cloves of garlic (minced)

1 1/2 teaspoons of fresh thyme

2 tablespoons of unsalted butter

1/2 cup of milk

1/4 cup of sour cream

1 1/2 teaspoons of salt

1/2 teaspoon of fresh ground black

pepper

Fried Chicken Recipe

5 lbs. chicken thighs (Debone thighs for easier eating. You may need to cut thighs in half to fit on top of "cupcakes")

1 tablespoon of salt

1/2 tablespoon of pepper

1 tablespoon of garlic powder

1/3 cup of corn starch

Vegetable oil for frying

INSTRUCTIONS

Cornbread Recipe

1. Preheat the oven to 350 degrees F.
2. In a medium-size bowl, mix the flour, baking soda, cornmeal, sugar, and salt.
3. In another medium-size bowl, mix the melted butter, eggs, and buttermilk.
4. Pour batter into cupcake liners and bake for 15-20 minutes or until an inserted toothpick comes out clean.

Garlic & Thyme Mashed Potato Recipe

1. Add olive oil to a medium-size pot and heat on medium-high.
2. Add garlic and thyme and sauté for 30 seconds, or until fragrant.
3. Add butter until melted.
4. Add the cooked potato, milk, sour cream, salt, and pepper.
5. Use an immersion blender or regular blender to puree the potato until smooth.
6. Pipe or scoop mashed potato onto each cornbread "cupcake."

Gravy

For the gravy, I took a shortcut and used an instant brown gravy packet. Follow packet instructions. Then drizzle about 2 teaspoons of gravy on top of the mashed potato.

Fried Chicken Recipe

5. Fill a medium-sized pot halfway with vegetable oil and heat on high.
6. In a large bowl, combine chicken, salt, pepper, and garlic powder. Toss until combined.
7. Add the cornstarch and toss until combined. Do not over toss as the corn starch will clump.
8. Fry the chicken in batches at 375 degrees F for 5 minutes or when wings float to the top with the desired color.
9. Remove the chicken and place on a plate lined with paper towels to remove the excess oil. Serve immediately.
10. Top each "cupcake" with a piece of fried chicken.

JAMAICAN JERK CHICKEN WINGS

This Jamaican Jerk Chicken Wings recipe is a great addition to any game-day, party, or just a regular wing craving. The jerk sauce ensures it's a party in your mouth. You can easily make it as hot as you can handle.

INGREDIENTS

20 Party-style chicken wings

1 Cup of Fresh Jerk marinade

1/4 Cup of Fresh Jerk marinade (for sauce)

2 Tablespoons of Ketchup

INSTRUCTIONS

1. Soak the pimento wood in some water for 20 minutes. Combine the Jerk Marinade and chicken wings in a large zip-top bag. Mix the marinade and wings together, ensuring that the chicken is completely covered. Close the bag and refrigerate for 4 hours to overnight (I strongly recommend overnight for an authentic taste).
2. Preheat an outdoor grill with coals.
3. Add the pimento wood that has been soaked for 20 mins. Place the wood directly on grates.
4. In a small saucepan, add the Ketchup and additional marinade. Stir to combine- simmer for about 10 minutes. Turn off heat and set aside.
5. Remove the chicken wings from the marinade and remove excess marinade. Cook the wings on the preheated grill, turning occasionally. Cook until the chicken is well browned and no longer pink, about 25 to 30 minutes.
6. Place grilled wings in a large bowl. Pour additional marinade over wings; toss to mix well. Serve with lime wedges. Enjoy!

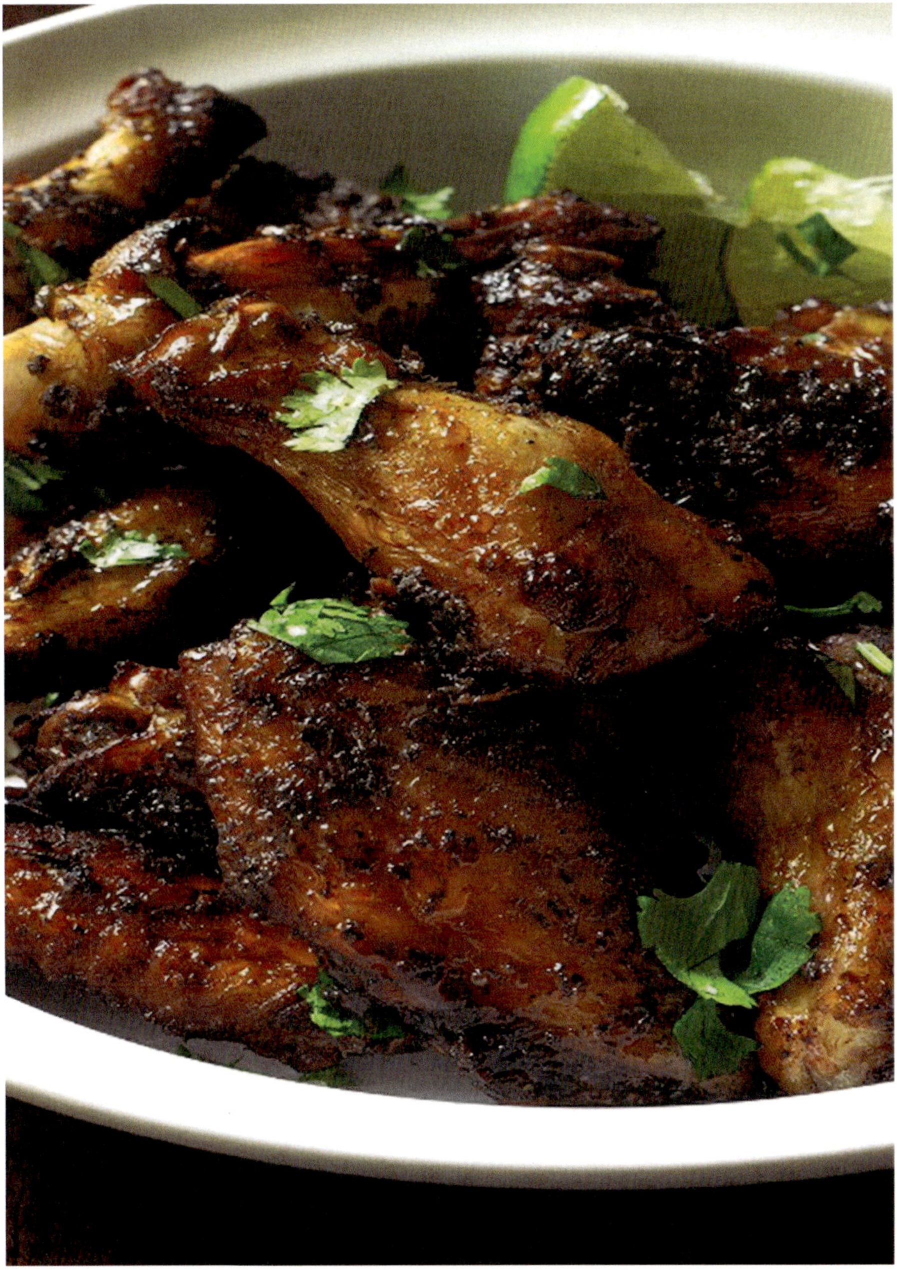

FRIED GOATS

Beef Tassot or Tassot Boeuf (Tassot Boeuf/Beef Tassot/Fried Beef Bits) is meat that has been marinated, boiled, and fried. It is part of what Haitians call "Fritaille," which is a mix of different types of fritters.

What is Tassot?

The word Tassot signifies the way the meat is cooked. It is typically served at parties, get-together, and even lunchtime or dinnertime. This dish is also sold at most Haitian restaurants.

You can make a tassot dish with any type of meat or poultry. The two common types of meat for tassot are beef and goat. It is also made with turkey, dark or white meat. This recipe is with beef.

How to make tassot the right way

What makes a tassot taste exquisite is the marinating time. You must allow the meat to marinate at least for 30 minutes or more with lemon juice, fresh herbs, and spices. The longer, the better.

You also have to let the meat cook in its marinade before adding water. If you add water before the meat even starts to cook in the pot, you will lose some of the flavors. You can also season the water as you add more to the pot. The best advice for cooking any type of meat is to never add cold water. Always add room temperature water of hot water to the pot to preserve the flavors.

Depending on the type of meat, or meat cuts, cooking time will be different. Goat meat takes a long time to cook. Goat meat Tassot is delicious, but patience is required. That is why more cooks prefer cooking Beef Tassot.

The best meat cuts for beef tassot

It is about what you can afford and how much time you have to cook. Beef Tassot is usually made with beef stew meat, filet mignon, tenderloin steak, or T-bone steak. The tender part of the beef is the loin, and one of the best meat cuts to make tassot.

What to serve tassot with

This dish is usually eaten with other fritters or as a meat dish with your meal. Because beef tends to be dry when cooked too long, a good sauce or gravy or even pikliz is required.

INGREDIENTS

3 lb. goat meat cubed

½ cup of sour orange juice

¼ cup of lime juice

Haitian epis/blended spices

1 teaspoon of hot pepper Habanero, preferably

1 tablespoon of salt

1 bouquet of garni Thyme and Parsley

1 tablespoon of parsley chopped

2 shallots chopped finely

4 cups of water

2 cups of oil if frying only

INSTRUCTIONS

1. Clean the meat very well and marinate for at least 2 hours or overnight with the Haitian epis/blended spices, sour orange juice, lime juice, hot pepper, and salt. Add meat to a pot and let boil first without adding any water. When the water starts to decrease, add 1 cup of water with bouquet garni, and add more water when necessary. More water may be needed for meat to be very tender. Remove meat from cooking liquid and set aside. Do not throw away cooking liquid: heat oil and fry pieces. Do not overcrowd the pan when frying.
2. Serve with a sauce prepared with 1 cup of cooking liquid, with chopped parsley, shallots, and additional chopped hot pepper. Serve hot.
3. If roasting in the oven, place pieces into a baking dish and roast until the meat is golden brown. It may take about 20 to 25 minutes. Drizzle meat with a little oil and fresh lemon juice prior to roasting. If roasting on a fire grill, drizzle with oil first.

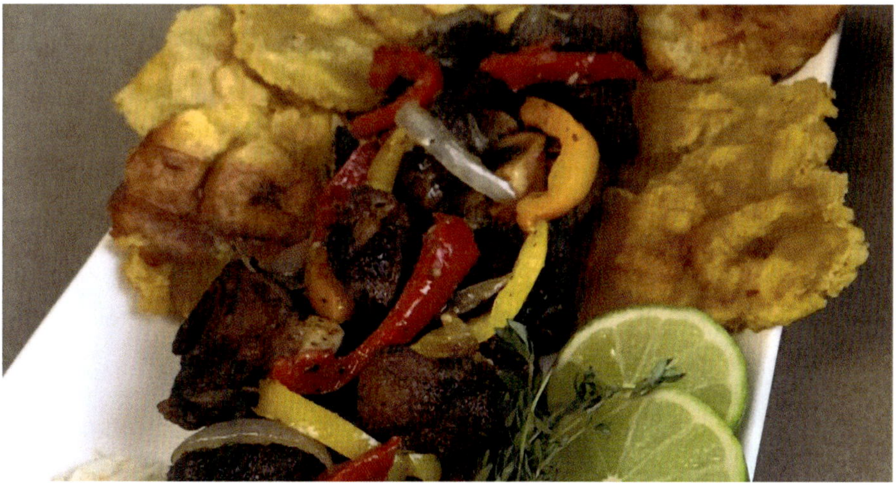

BAKED JERK CHICKEN

It's a lot easier to make Jerk Chicken at home than you think. The trick to making oven-baked jerk chicken is to marinate it overnight, then broil it in the oven for a crispy caramelized skin.

The flavor comes from the marinate, which is the perfect combination of sweet and spicy. Sweet from the molasses and spicy from the habanero.

How to make Baked Jerk Chicken

- *Marinate:* Add oil, molasses, lime juice, habanero peppers, ginger, garlic, and spices to a food processor and pulse until combined. Reserve 1/4 cup of the marinade, set aside. Pour the rest of the marinade into a large zip lock bag along with the chicken. Marinate for at least an hour or preferably overnight.
- *Bake:* When you are ready to cook, preheat the oven to 350 degrees. Take the chicken out of the marinade and place the chicken in a cast-iron skillet or oven-safe pan. Cook for 1 hour or until chicken is fully cooked. Take out of the oven and brush on the reserved marinade.
- *Broil chicken:* Turn oven to broil and cook for 3-4 minutes or until the skin is browned and crispy. (Make sure to keep a close eye on it, so it does not burn.)
- *Serve:* Immediately with fresh chopped cilantro and lime wedges for serving.

Tips for making The Best Baked Jerk Chicken

- Don't skip the marinating. It makes the chicken super tender and adds so much flavor. The longer you marinate the chicken, the better!
- I recommend using chicken thighs or drumsticks in this recipe. They have more fat and will keep the chicken from drying out.
- If you can't find habanero peppers, you can substitute scotch bonnets. Just adjust to taste. Scotch bonnets tend to be a bit spicier.

INGREDIENTS

¼ c. vegetable oil

2 tbsp. of molasses

Juice of 1 lime

1 habanero pepper, stemmed and seeded

6 green onions

1 (1-inch) chunk fresh ginger

5 garlic cloves

1 tbsp. of thyme

1½ tsp. of all spice

¼ tsp. of cardamom

1 tsp. of salt

¼ tsp. of pepper

2-3 lbs. of chicken thighs, drumsticks, or wings (skin-on)

1 lime, sliced

INSTRUCTIONS

1. Preheat the oven to 325 degrees.
2. In the bowl of a food processor or blender, add the vegetable oil, molasses, lime juice, habanero, green onions, ginger, garlic cloves, thyme, allspice, cardamom, salt, and pepper. Process until smooth. The mixture will be fairly thick, almost pesto-like.
3. Add chicken to a large sauté pan or Dutch oven (with a lid). Pour or brush the mixture over the chicken, reserving about ¼ c. for the final broil. Add lime slices. Cover and bake for 2 to 2½ hours.
4. Brush the chicken with the reserved coating and broil uncovered until charred, about 5 minutes or so, depending on your broil setting. Serve immediately.

Notes

The habanero doesn't really add crazy heat to this recipe; next time, I'd add two!

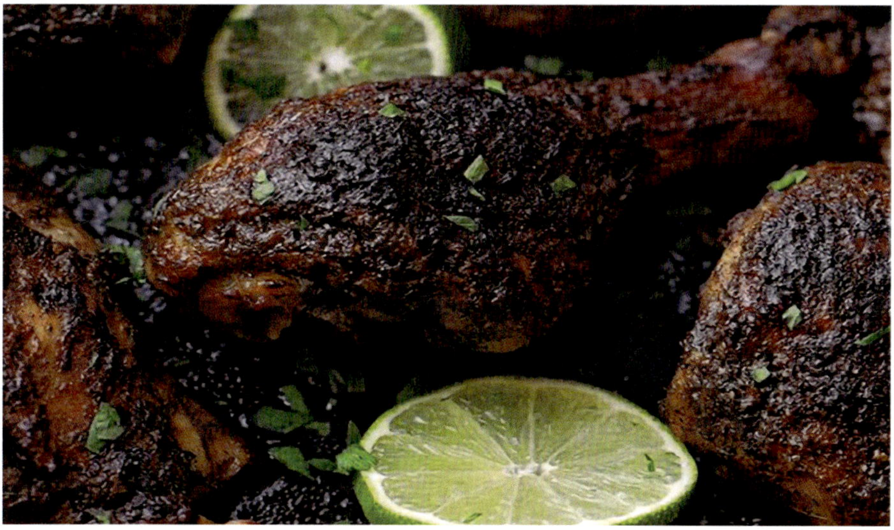

LAMB CHOPS WITH MINT JELLY

This Jamaican Jerk Chicken Wings recipe is a great addition to any game-day, party, or just a regular wing craving. The jerk sauce ensures it's a party in your mouth. You can easily make it as hot as you can handle.

INGREDIENTS

For the rub

3 tablespoons of Salt

2 tablespoons of Domino® Golden Sugar

2 tablespoons of Garlic powder

1 tablespoon of cracked black pepper

1 teaspoon of dried rosemary leaves

1 teaspoon of onion powder

1 teaspoon of Dried mint

1 teaspoon of parsley flakes

For the lamb chops

2 racks Lamb, frenched and clean from most fat

2 tablespoons of Vegetable oil

2 tablespoons of unsalted butter

5 sprigs of fresh rosemary

2 cloves of Garlic

INSTRUCTIONS

1. Mix all the ingredients of the rub. Cut the lamb racks into 2 half-racks and season the lamb generously with the rub. Set on a plate and let rest for 25 minutes at room temperature.
2. Heat oil in a large skillet over medium-high heat. Lay the lamb racks in the pan, fat side down. Brown the lamb while occasionally turning with thongs until all sides are golden brown. Reduce the heat to medium and add butter, 3 sprigs of rosemary, and garlic to the skillet. Continue cooking, basting the lamb with butter, and occasionally turning until the lamb's internal temperature is 130°F for medium. Remove lamb from heat and allow resting for 5 minutes. Cut the lamb chops and serve. Garnish the plate with fresh rosemary sprigs.

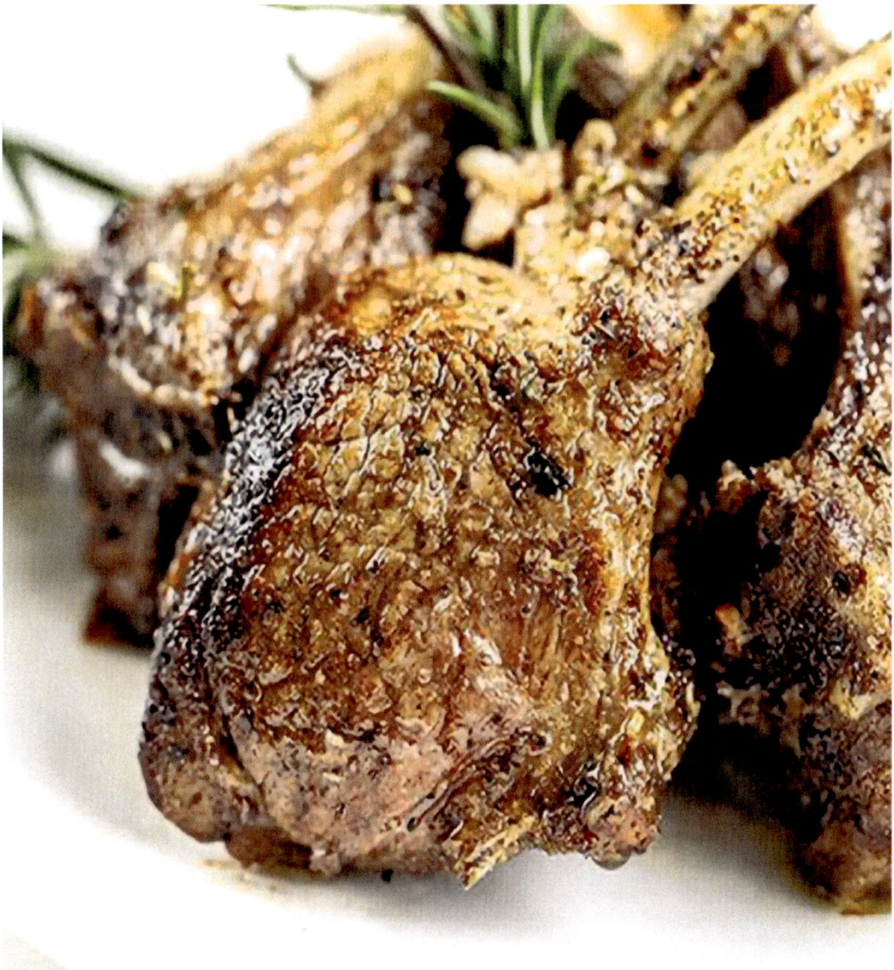

SPINACH PESTO, FETA, AND SHRIMP

INGREDIENTS

For the spinach pesto:

- 1 cup of baby spinach (packed)
- 2 tablespoons of dill
- 2 tablespoons of parsley
- 1 green onion
- 1 clove of garlic
- 2 tablespoons of walnuts, toasted
- 1/4 cup of parmigiano reggiano (parmesan), grated
- 3 tablespoons of olive oil
- 1/2 lemon, juice, and zest
- salt and pepper to taste
- For the shrimp, souvlaki:1 pound of large shrimp, shelled and deveined
- 2 cloves of garlic, chopped
- 1 lemon, juice, and zest
- 1 tablespoon of yogurt
- 1/4 cup of olive oil
- 1 teaspoon of oregano
- 1/4 teaspoon of salt
- 1/4 teaspoon of pepper

For the spinach pesto, feta, and shrimp tortellini:

- 1 pound of cheese tortellini
- 1/2 cup of feta, crumbled
- 2 green onions, thinly sliced
- 1 tablespoon of dill, chopped
- 1 tablespoon of parsley, chopped

INSTRUCTIONS

1. For the spinach pesto: Puree everything in a food processor until smooth.
2. For the shrimp: Marinate the shrimp in the mixture of the remaining ingredients for 30 minutes to overnight before cooking in a pan or grilling over medium-high heat until cooked, about 2-3 minutes per side.
3. For the spinach pesto, feta and shrimp tortellini: Cook the tortellini as directed before tossing it with the pesto, feta and shrimp and herbs and enjoying!

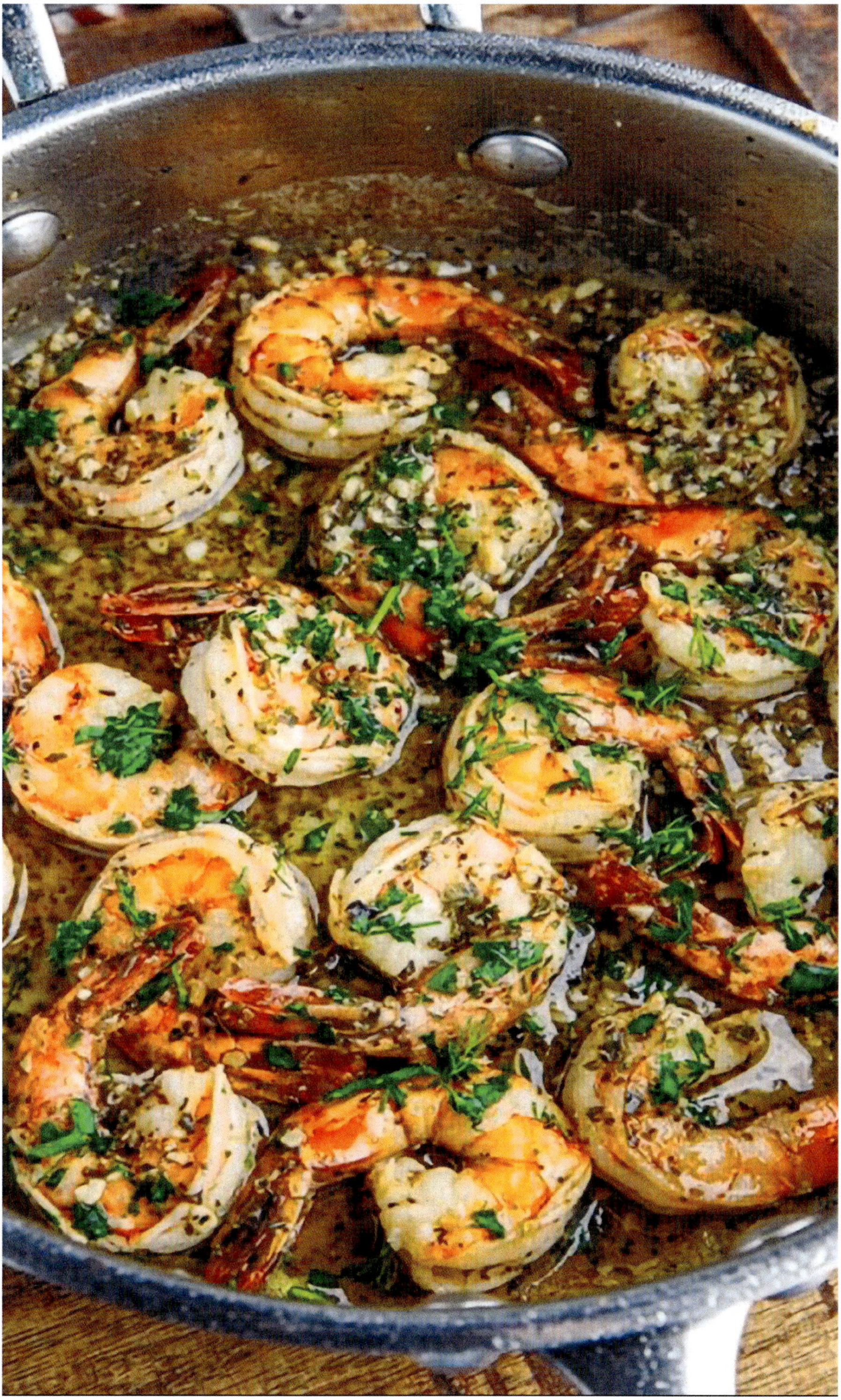

07
DESSERTS

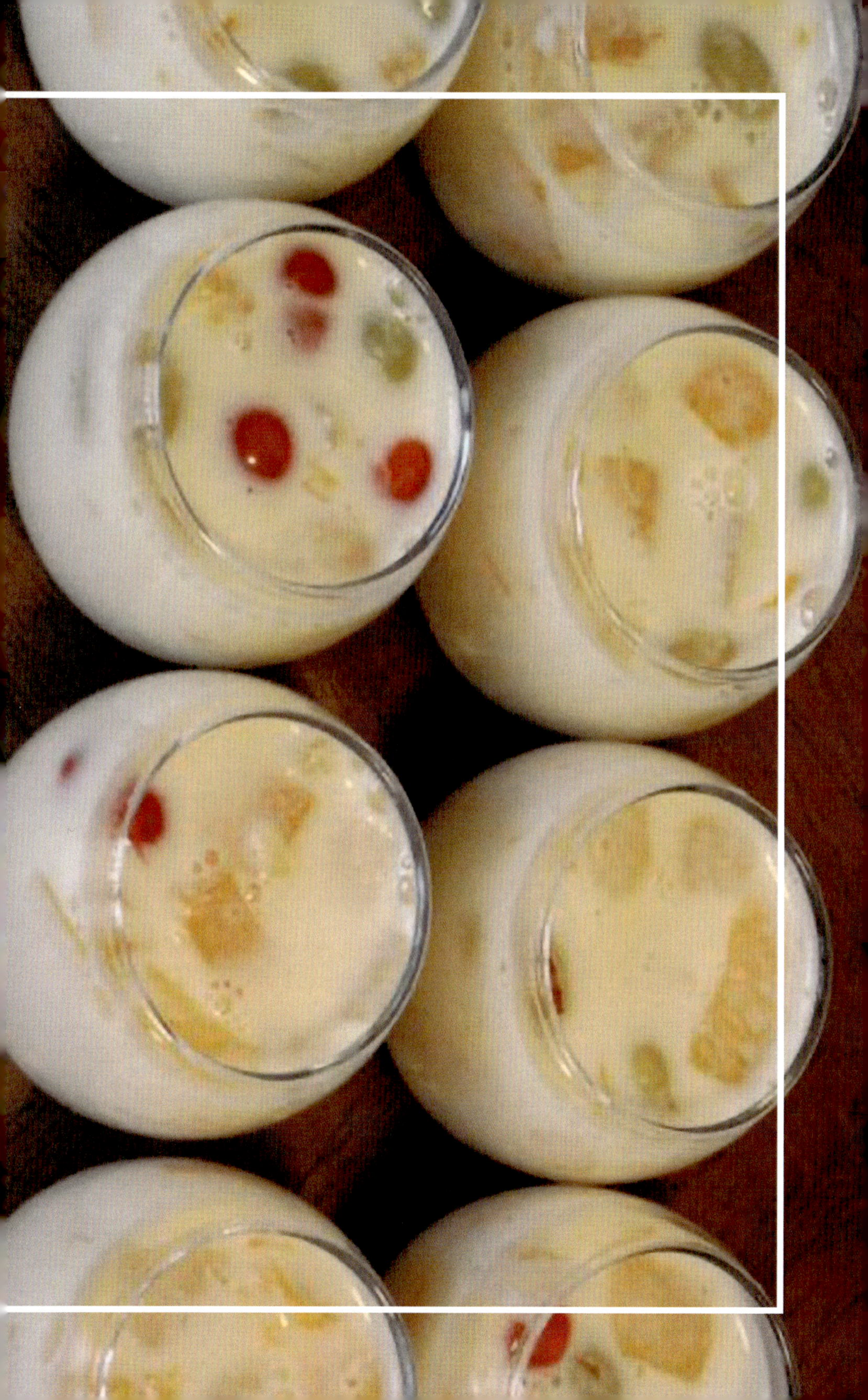

CORNMEAL PUDDING

Tell me if there is a better way to kick start the day than with a warm, hearty breakfast. If you wake up wanting something a bit sweet to combat early morning cravings, then you are in luck. This Jamaican cornmeal porridge will do just that.

What I like about it is that it's so filling and very energizing, making it ideal for a pick me up in the a.m. breakfast.

Caribbean breakfast dish that dates back more than a century.

It's made with yellow cornmeal, infused with earthy spices like cinnamon and nutmeg. Most often, condensed coconut milk is added for a rich and sweet taste.

An incredible cross between traditional porridge and grits. You have sweetness along with the warmth from the cinnamon, nutmeg, as well as the sweet "corny" flavor of the cornmeal itself.

A hot cereal with depth and texture that is not too heavy on the stomach. It Tastes great on its own, but when combined with fruits and nuts, it's heavenly. My favorite is mango and blueberries.

You can't go wrong with sliced banana, mango, slivered almonds, and/or walnuts. Lastly, you can serve this for brunch, lunch, dinner, or an indulgent snack.

INGREDIENTS

1/2 cup of finely ground cornmeal

2 1/2 cups of water (divided)

1 (3-inch) cinnamon stick

Sugar and milk to taste

INSTRUCTIONS

1. To a medium bowl, add cornmeal and 1/2 cup of water. Stir and let stand undisturbed to soak for 5 minutes.
2. While the cornmeal is soaking, add the remaining 2 cups of water to a medium saucepan along with the cinnamon stick. Cover and bring to a boil.
3. When the water is boiling, pour in soaked cornmeal as well as any liquid in the bowl to the saucepan. Lower the heat to a simmer and whisk to avoid lumps.
4. Cook covered for 15 to 20 minutes.
5. Remove the pot from the heat, sweeten with sugar and milk to taste, stirring until fully incorporated. Serve hot in heated bowls if desired.

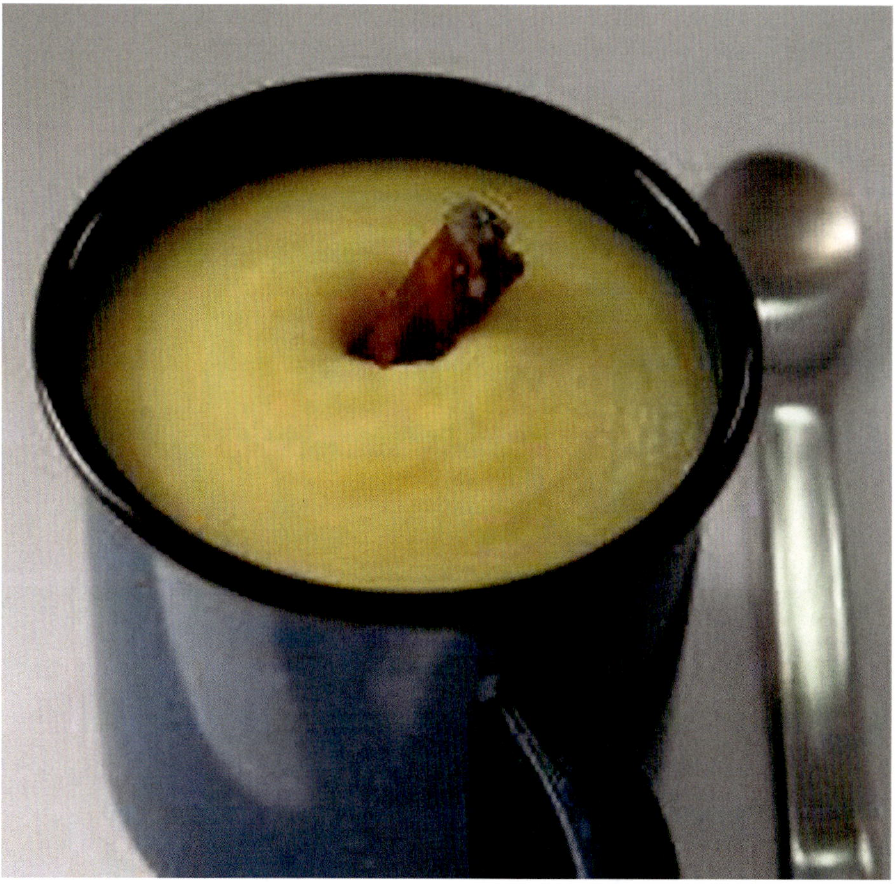

MINI APPLE PIES

These are so easy and quick. You've just got to give them a try! Plantains are super budget-friendly too- so there's really no reason not to go for it!

INGREDIENTS

8 cups of apples, cut into 1/2 inch bits

12 tablespoons of flour

1 1/2 cups of sugar

4 heaping teaspoons of cinnamon

1/4-1/2 teaspoon of nutmeg (depending on how much you like nutmeg, you could also leave it out)

4 tablespoons of chilled butter cut into 24 equal portions.

2 boxes of pie crusts (four chilled NOT frozen crusts)

INSTRUCTIONS

1. Mix the apples with the flour, sugar, and cinnamon.
2. Unroll your first pie crust, and cut several circles out. Continue this until you have enough crusts. I found that a wide mouth mason jar ring worked perfectly. Line each cup of your muffin tin with a tiny pie crust.
3. Gently fill the crusts with your apple mixture; you should be able to fill until slightly mounded; put a dab of butter on each pie. Cover as desired with leftover dough. Brush with melted butter and bake at 400 degrees Fahrenheit for 18 to 22 minutes.

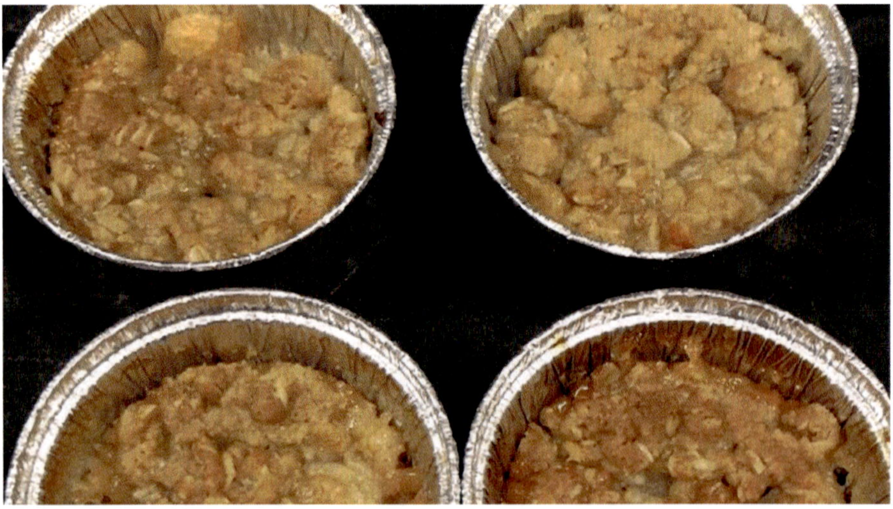

COCONUT SUGAR CARAMELIZED PLANTAINS

These are so easy and quick. You've just got to give them a try! Plantains are super budget-friendly too- so there's really no reason not to go for it!

INGREDIENTS

3 ripe plantains (tender to the touch and yellow going on brown)

3 tbsp of coconut sugar (or sub cane sugar)

1/4 tsp of ground cinnamon

1 pinch sea salt

1-2 Tbsp of coconut oil

Coconut Whipped Cream

INSTRUCTIONS

1. Heat a large cast-iron or metal skillet over medium-high heat and chop your plantains in 1/2-inch slices.
2. Add to a mixing bowl and toss with coconut sugar, cinnamon, and sea salt.
3. Once the skillet is hot, add coconut oil and only as many plantains as will fit comfortably in the pan without crowding. Cook for 2-3 minutes on each side or until browned and caramelized.
4. Serve warm with dairy-free ice cream or coconut whipped cream. Best when fresh, though leftovers will keep in the fridge covered for a few days.

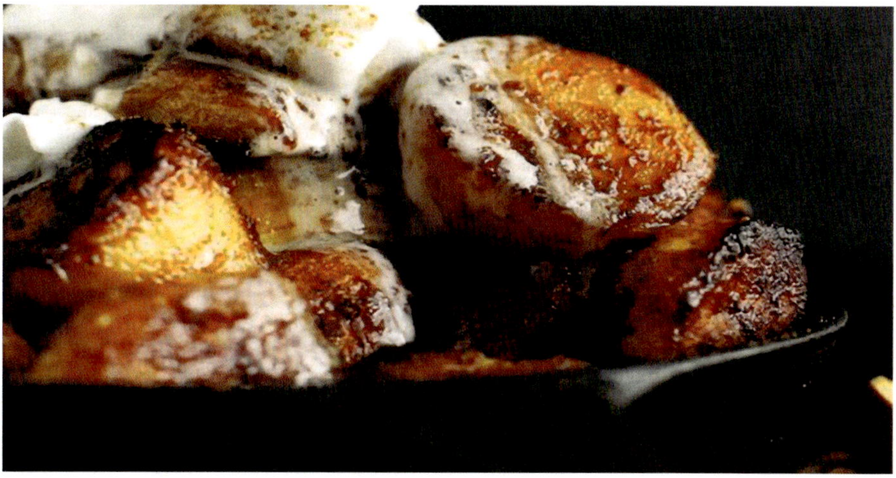

PINEAPPLE UPSIDE-DOWN CAKE

When baking an upside-down pineapple cake, a basic cake recipe is usually ideal, and whatever spices or extract you wish to add to make the cake more flavorful is always good to do. The cake can be baked perfectly, and you can even remove it from the pan immediately as it is usually done.

INGREDIENTS

- Nonstick cooking spray or butter for 10-inch round pan
- 1 cup of unsalted butter 2 sticks
- 1 cup of sugar
- 2 cups of flour sifted
- 2 teaspoons of baking powder
- 3 eggs at room temperature
- ¾ cup of pineapple juice
- 1 teaspoon of vanilla
- ¾ to 1 cup of brown sugar
- 1 – 20 ounces of pineapple or fresh pineapple can be sliced
- 1 tablespoon of dark rum
- Cherries
- Dried Prunes

INSTRUCTIONS

1. Preheat the oven to 350 degrees F. Spray 10-inch round cake pan with nonstick cooking spray and coat with flour.
2. In a large bowl, beat butter and sugar at medium speed with an electric mixer until creamy. Add the eggs, 1 at a time, beating well after each addition. Stir in the vanilla, rum, and pineapple juice.
3. Gradually add sifted flour mixed with baking powder and stir to incorporate
4. Use additional butter or nonstick spray to prepare the pan. Add brown sugar to the prepared pan. Arrange the pineapple slices, prunes, and cherries over the brown sugar. Reserve remaining pineapple slices and cherries for another use. Pour batter into the pan and spread evenly. Bake in the oven at 350 degrees for about 40 minutes or until the tester inserted into the center comes out clean. Turn the cake out onto a platter and serve at room temperature.
5. Yield 10 to 12 servings

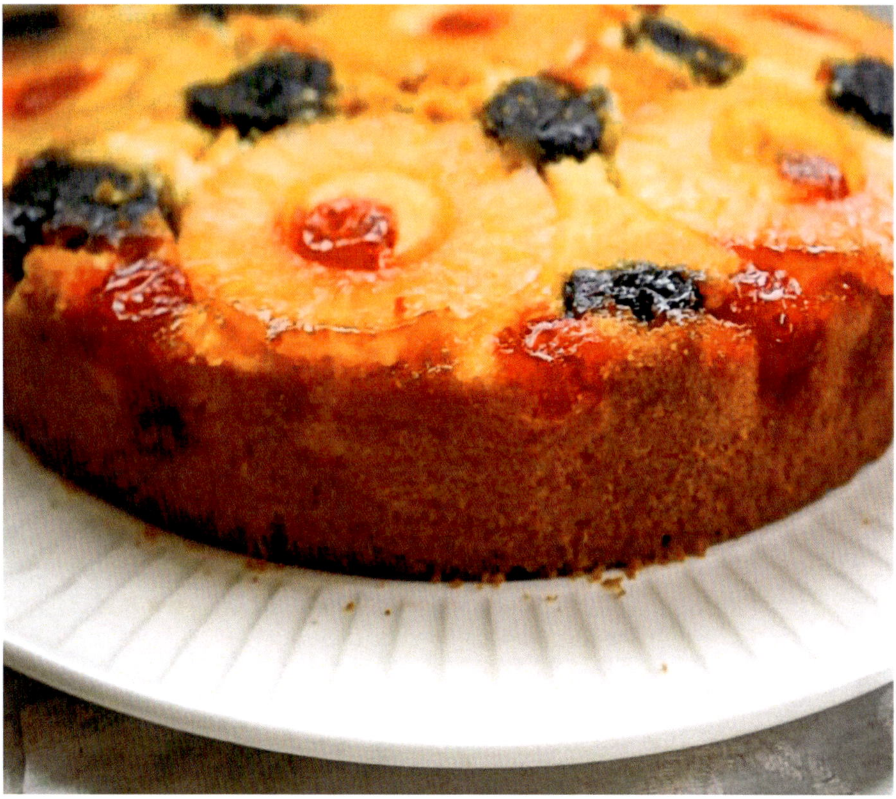

GRILLED PINEAPPLE WITH CINNAMON SUGAR

Sweet caramelized grilled pineapple with cinnamon sugar is a healthy, fat-free dessert that is fast and easy to make. This simple dessert is frequently served in Brazilian Steakhouses, but you can make it at home. Grilled pineapple will not burn your mouth, eat as much as you want.

If you have ever been to a Brazilian Steakhouse, you have probably seen the grilled pineapple on their rotisserie. It is a common flavor combination in Brazilian cuisine. This Grilled Pineapple recipe only takes 20 minutes to start to finish and is a sweet, tangy, juicy dream!

Serve this Grilled Pineapple as an easy appetizer, side, or even dessert all summer long. I've included tips on how to choose pineapple, how to cut pineapple, how to grill outdoors, and how to grill indoors so you can enjoy this Grilled Pineapple year round!

INGREDIENTS

1 pineapple

1/2 cup of brown sugar

1 tablespoon of cinnamon

INSTRUCTIONS

1. Get the grill ready. Coat the grill with cooking spray and preheat to medium heat. (or pre-heat an indoor grilling pan).
2. Slice the top and bottom off of the pineapple, then trim off the outer skin, cut out any brown "eyes," and slice it into spears. (You do not have to remove the center core if you don't want to, the core will get soft and sweet when it grills, and you can eat it.)
3. Combine the brown sugar and cinnamon in a bowl then sprinkle it on the pineapple spears.
4. Grill for 4 to 5 minutes on each side or until golden brown and caramelized.

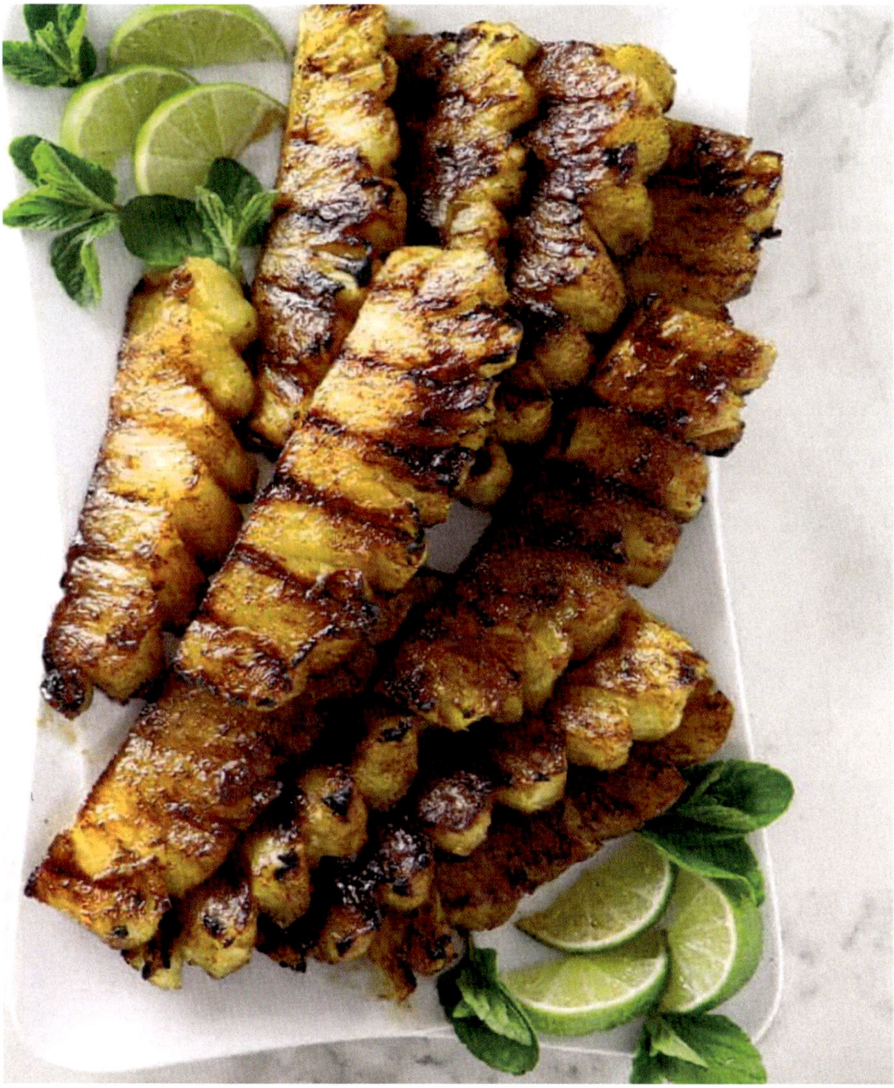

HAITIAN DESSERT BLAN MANJE

"This Haitian Dessert is a delicious blend of island flavors. The base is coconut with surprise fruit blends of cherry, pineapple, and other great island flavors. This dish is really quick and easy to make and is a great way to surprise and delight at any event. This is a Haitian Coconut Fruit cocktail that you can even spice up by adding some rum or vodka for a treat very similar to the classic Haitian drink Cremas."

These are so easy and quick. You've just got to give them a try! Plantains are super budget-friendly too- so there's really no reason not to go for it!

INGREDIENTS

1 Can Evaporated Milk

1 Can Condensed Milk

1 Can Coconut Milk

1 Can Fruit Cocktail

Vanilla Extract

Coconut Extract

2 packs of Gelatin

1/4 Cup of Hot Water

Pinch of Salt

INSTRUCTIONS

1. Mix the can of evaporated milk, condensed milk, and coconut milk together.
2. Add the can of fruit cocktail
3. Add vanilla and coconut extract and a pinch of salt
4. Now make the gelatin mixture: mix 2 packs of gelatin with a 1/4 cup of hot water–not boiling
5. Mix well, then add gelatin mixture to the milk mixture, all the while mixing.
6. Refrigerate for at least 4 hours before enjoying

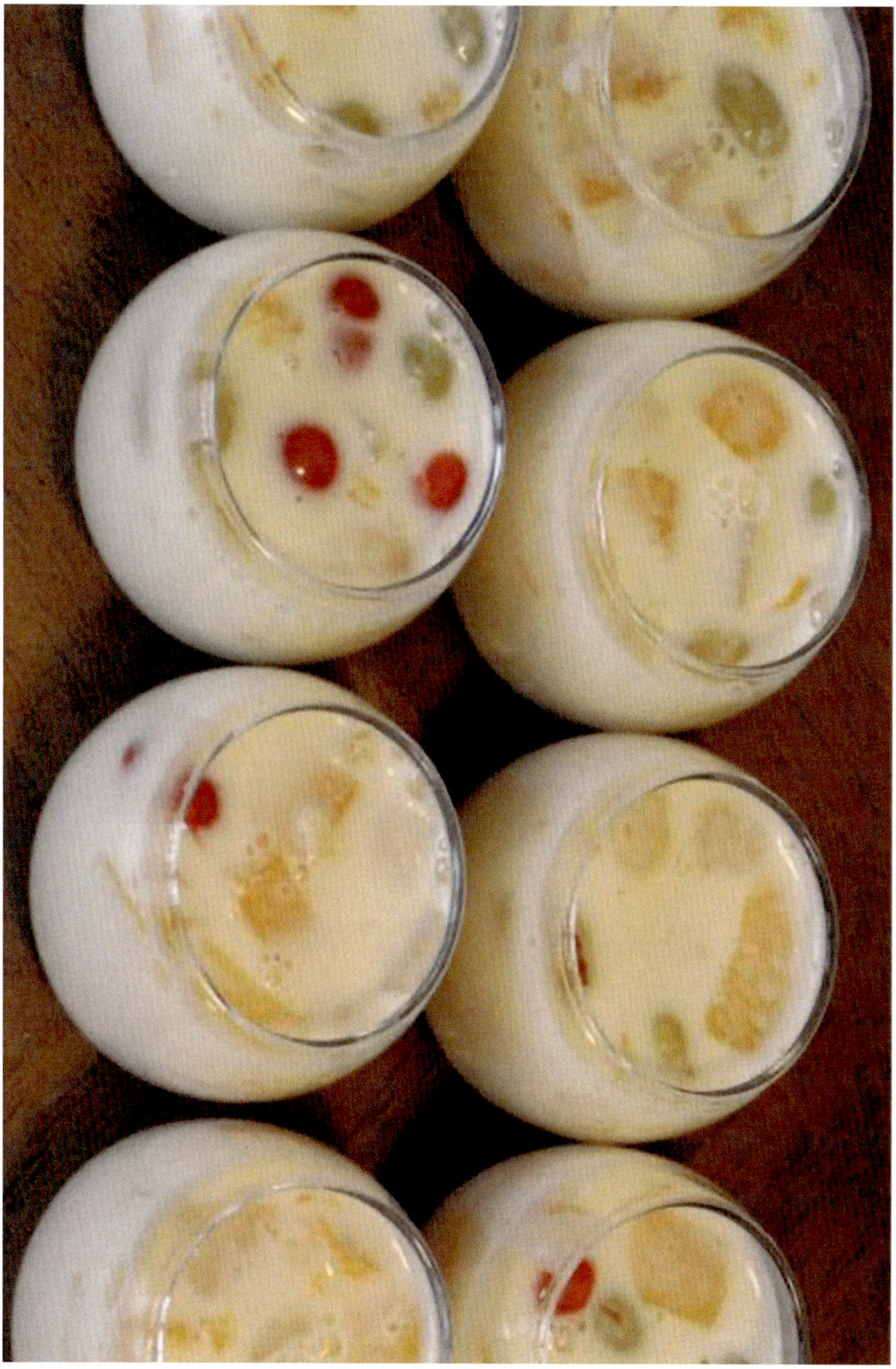

PUMPKIN SPICE LATTE RECIPE

EASY. We're talking of 6 fridge and pantry staple ingredients – pumpkin puree, pumpkin pie spice, sugar, milk (any kind,) vanilla, and coffee or espresso – combined to make a cozy, homemade drink in less than 5 minutes.

Customizable. Don't have an espresso machine? No problem. Use strongly-brewed coffee instead, which, spoiler alert: I might like better than the espresso version!

Cheap. Think spending $5-7 on a coffee shop's PSL, sounds insane? That's because IT IS!

Low(er) in sugar. I did some calculating – a short, nonfat, no whip Pumpkin Spice Latte from Starbucks has 24 grams of sugar. That's crazy and not just because nobody orders a short, nonfat, no whip PSL from Starbucks, right? The at-home version has less than 13 grams of sugar.

Kid-friendly. If your child wants in on a little pumpkin spice action like Mom and Dad, give it to him or her with this warm drink made without espresso or coffee. Lincoln went bananas for it and has asked for a mug every single day since Friday! 2 cups of milk (dairy or non-dairy)

INGREDIENTS

2 tablespoons of pumpkin puree

1 to 3 tablespoons of sugar, depending on how sweet you like it

1 tablespoon of vanilla extract

1/2 teaspoon of pumpkin pie spice, plus more for serving

1/2 cup of strong hot coffee

INSTRUCTIONS

1. Whipped cream, for serving
2. Add milk, pumpkin puree, and sugar to a saucepan over medium heat. Heat until hot, but do not boil. Remove the saucepan from the heat and whisk in the vanilla, pumpkin pie spice, and the coffee.

3. Divide the mixture between two mugs. Top with whipped cream and a sprinkle of pumpkin pie spice.

- Milk: This taste best with 2% or whole milk, but you can substitute with skim milk. Non-dairy milk like soy, almond, or coconut milk will also work.
- Sugar: This recipe calls for 1 to 3 tablespoons of sugar. How much you use is up to you. We tend to prefer less sugar in our drinks. You can also use a sugar substitute. Add this to taste.
- Pumpkin Pie Spice Blend: Find pumpkin pie spice at the store or make it at home. You likely have everything you need to make it already. Mix the following spices in a spice jar: 1 1/2 tablespoons ground cinnamon + 2 teaspoons of ground ginger + 1/2 teaspoon of ground nutmeg + a pinch of ground cloves.
- More Pumpkin Flavor: Since posting this recipe, some readers have noted that they would prefer a stronger pumpkin flavor. You can achieve these two ways: increase the puree by 1 to 2 tablespoons or cook a large batch of puree down in a saucepan over medium heat until reduced and concentrated in flavor, and then use in the latte.

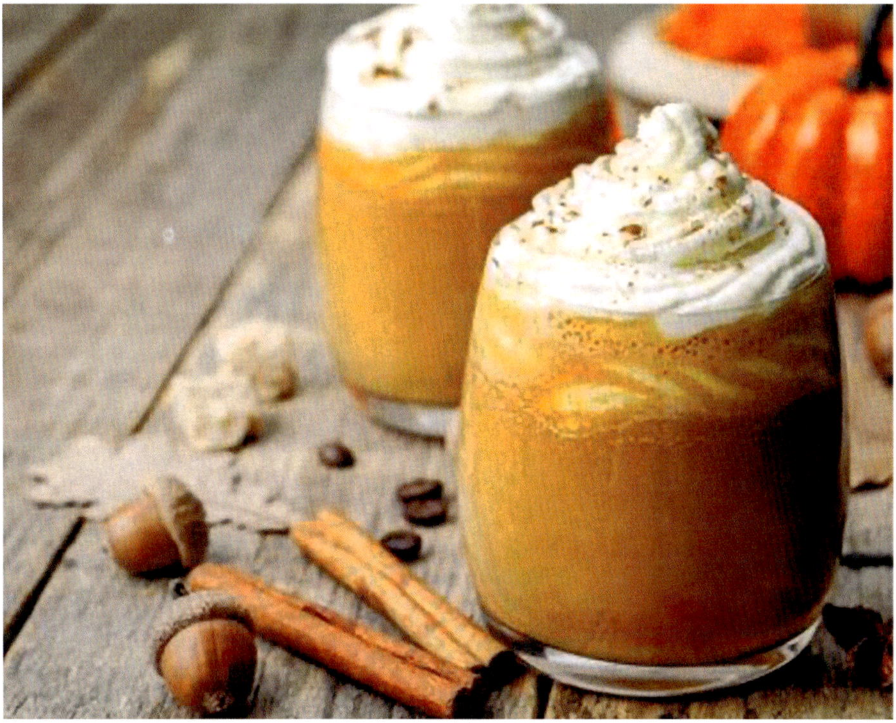

LABOUYI BANNANN/ PLANTAIN PORIN

One of the many foods Haitians eat for breakfast is Labouyi Bannann (Plantain Porridge). It's porridge, essentially– one made from ripe banana and unripe plantain.

There are myriad ways to spell it, but only one way to eat it– with a spoon. Make that two ways to eat it hot or cold. Either way, it's a good way to start the day.

Porridges have long been an integral part of Caribbean cuisine. Porridge is meant to fortify and strengthen for long periods of time. Unlike typical porridges, which use grains such as oats, wheat, and corn, Labouyi uses plantains. The porridge is sweet and creamy with the consistency of light grits. Labouyi can also be made with flour and cornmeal. Try starting the day off with it.

You can't go wrong with sliced banana, mango, slivered almonds, and/or walnuts. Lastly, you can serve this for brunch, lunch, dinner, or an indulgent snack.

INGREDIENTS

- 1 Green Plantain (Washed)
- 3 cups of water
- 1 Star Anise
- 1/2 cup of Evaporated Milk
- 1/2 cup of Coconut Milk
- 1/2 tsp of cinnamon Powder of 1 stick
- 1/4 cup of sugar
- 1 Tbsp of butter
- 1 tsp of vanilla extract
- 1 tsp of salt (or to taste)

INSTRUCTIONS

1. Peel the skin of the plantain and cut into small 4-8 small pieces. It is ok to leave some of the skin for extra nutrients.
2. In a blender, puree the plantain and 2 cups of water.
3. In a 1-quart saucepan, add 1 cup of water, evaporated milk, coconut milk, cinnamon, star anise and bring to boil.

4. Once the pot is boiling, add the plantain puree to the pot and bring to a boil while stirring continuously for 5 min. The porridge will thicken slightly.
5. Add the salt, sugar, vanilla, and keep stirring for 10 min.
6. Reduce the heat to medium and keep stirring for another 10 min while tasting porridge to ensure the plantain is thoroughly cooked. The porridge is ready when the texture is creamy.
7. Serve warm with some Haitian Bread.

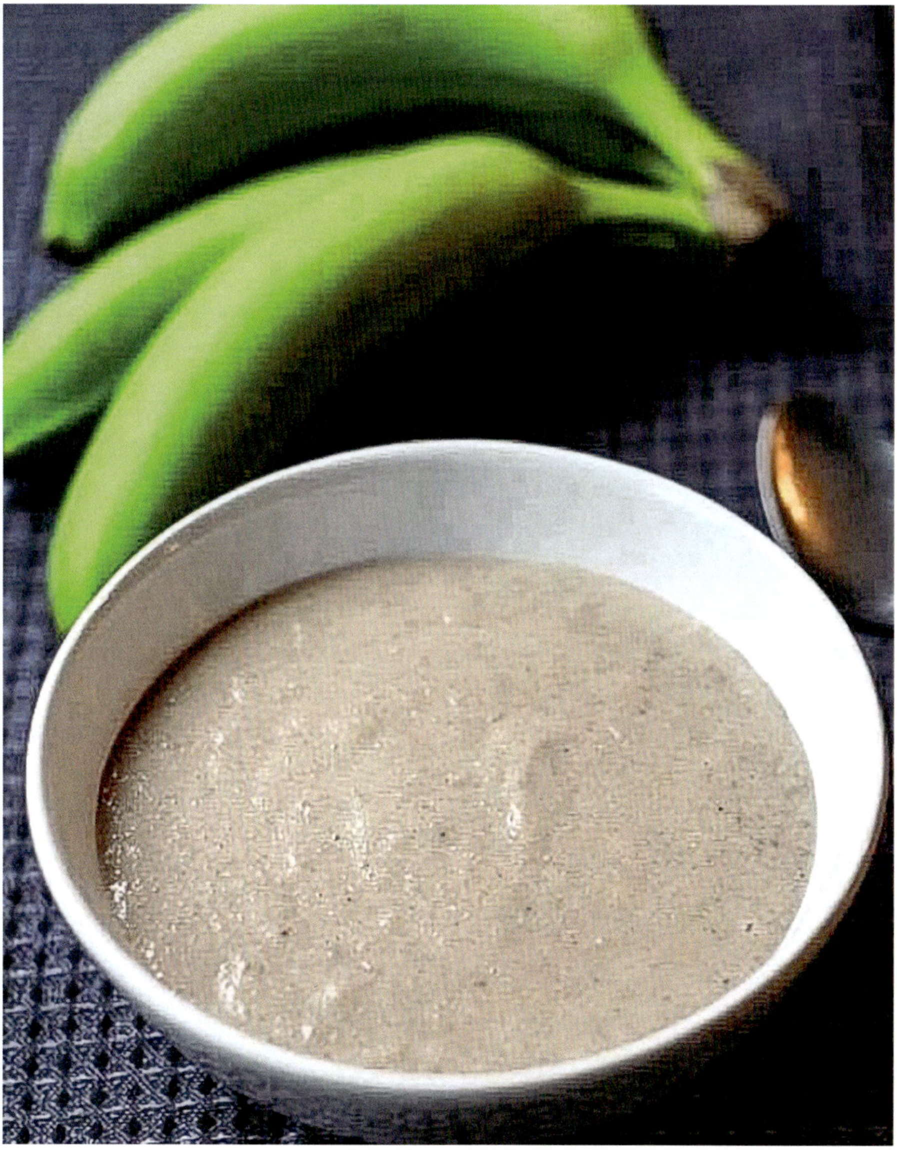

TROPICAL PINEAPPLE-COCONUT SMOOTHIE

This simple and flavorful 3-ingredient tropical smoothie is bursting with pineapple and coconut flavors. A fun and fruity drink, perfect for any time of the day, morning, noon, or night! Breakfast, snack, post-workout, you name it!

INGREDIENTS

- 2 cups of frozen pineapple chunks
- 1 cup of frozen mango chunks
- ¾ cup of FAGE Total 5%, 2%, or 0%
- ½ cup of pineapple juice
- ½ cup of canned coconut milk
- ¼ tsp of vanilla extract
- Toasted coconut flakes, optional

INSTRUCTIONS

1. In a blender, combine pineapple, mango, FAGE Total, pineapple juice, coconut milk, and vanilla. Blend until smooth.
2. Divide between two chilled glasses. If desired, garnish with coconut flakes. Serve immediately.

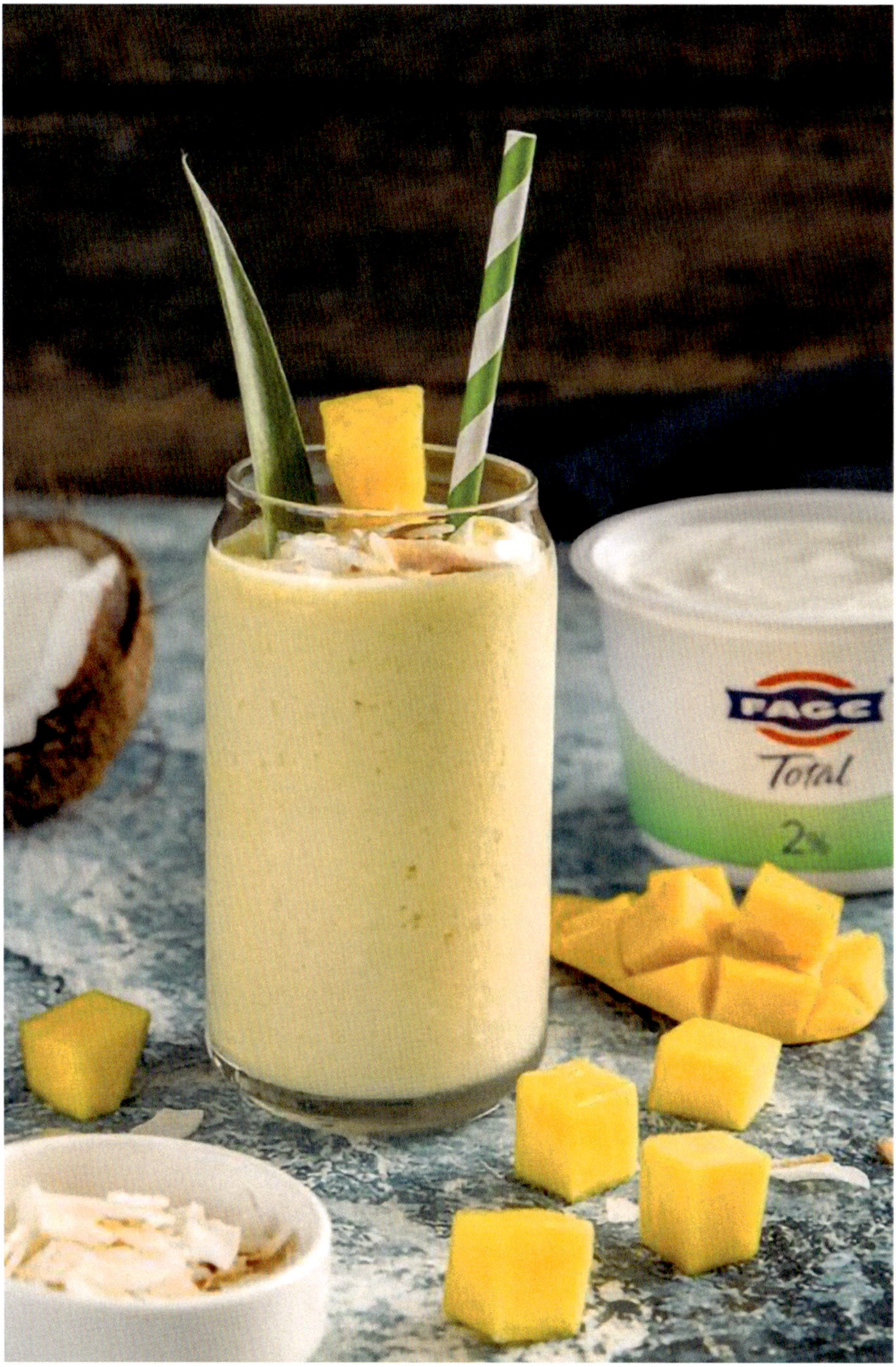
FAGE
Total
2%

TROPICAL JACKFRUIT SMOOTHIE

Frozen mango and frozen banana help to thicken this smoothie. If you substitute fresh fruits, the smoothie will be a lot looser.

Full fat canned coconut milk makes this jackfruit smoothie super-rich and creamy. For a lighter version, substitute in light coconut milk or coconut water.

If you cannot find fresh jackfruit, canned RIPE jackfruit will work. However, the resulting smoothie will be A LOT sweeter. Canned jackfruit is packaged in a sweet syrup.

This can be served for breakfast, as a snack, or as a mocktail option. If you want to booze it up, go ahead and add a shot of rum and turn this into a jackfruit pinna colada!

INGREDIENTS

- 7 pieces fresh jackfruit
- 1/4 cup of frozen banana slices
- 1/2 cup of frozen mango chunks
- 1/2 cup of well-shaken canned coconut milk, unsweetened
- 1/3 cup of pineapple juice

INSTRUCTIONS

1. Fresh banana and mango can also be used in place of frozen. However, the resulting smoothie will not be as thick.
2. Coconut milk makes this rich and creamy. You can also substitute in coconut water for a lighter beverage.

Want to make this into a cocktail?

1. Add 1 1/2 oz of dark or light rum when blending all the ingredients. It turns into a jackfruit pinna colada!

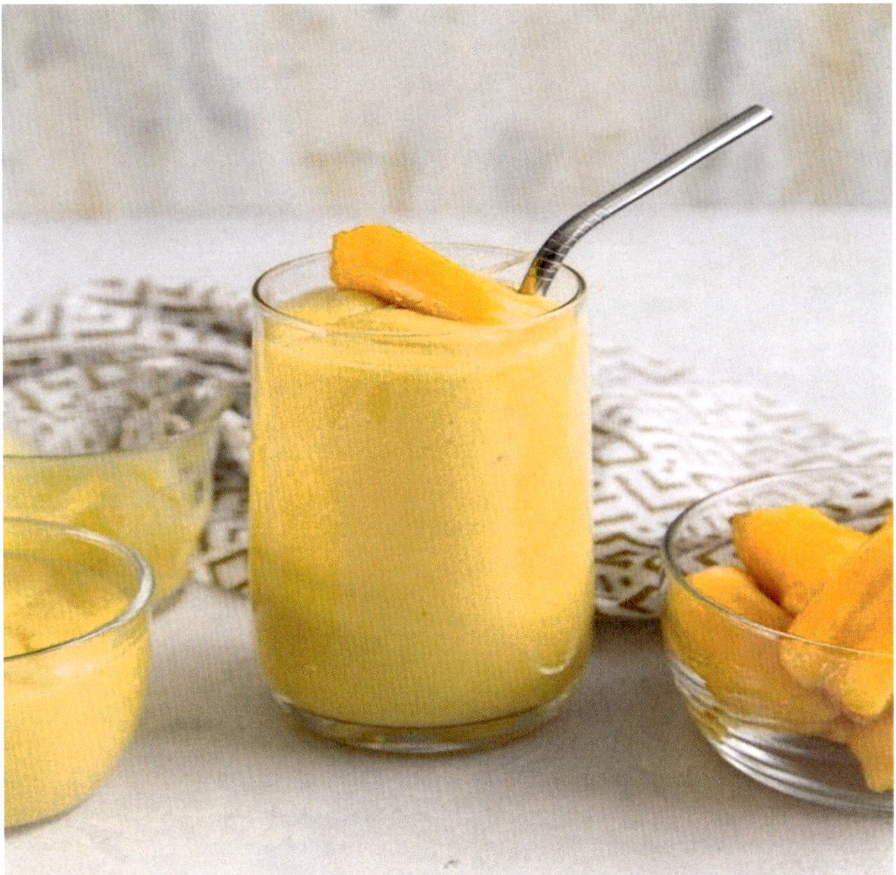

Made in United States
Orlando, FL
04 November 2026

90207200R00119